AF400016

Maher Asaad Baker

Raising Warriors

Contents

Introduction 1

Mental Strength 8

Leading by Example 45

Communication.. 72

Clear Boundaries... 96

Problem-Solving Skills 124

Independence and Self-Reliance........................ 152

Gratitude and Positivity 175

Physical Health.. 193

Supporting Your Child 216

Challenges and Setbacks.................................... 234

Age-Specific Strategies...................................... 263

Digital Age 290

Disclaimer.. 319

About the Author 321

Introduction

The importance of self-discipline and boundaries in the development of young people is crucial. These aspects play a significant role in shaping a child's behavior and preparing them for success in various aspects of life.

Self-discipline, also known as self-restraint or self-determination, refers to the ability to control one's thoughts, feelings, and actions to achieve one's goals. It is a valuable skill that helps children make responsible decisions, resist temptation, and persevere in the face of challenges.

On the other hand, boundaries define the limits and rules set by caregivers and guardians to create a safe and nurturing environment in which children can thrive. They help children understand their rights and responsibilities, build self-respect, and develop healthy and beneficial relationships.

Self-discipline is like a muscle that needs regular exercise and reinforcement to grow and improve. Children who learn self-discipline from a young age are more likely to succeed in their academic pursuits, social interactions, and emotional well-being. They can focus their attention, control their impulses, and manage their emotions effectively, which are essential skills for achieving long-term goals and navigating life's challenges.

Self-discipline empowers children to prioritize their efforts, maintain order and structure, and meet deadlines, all of which are essential habits for academic and professional success. Additionally, it instills in children a strong work ethic, resilience, and the ability to bounce back from adversities and setbacks.

Boundaries provide children with a sense of stability, predictability, and structure in their lives. When caregivers and guardians establish clear and consistent boundaries, children experience a secure and understandable environment, fostering a positive sense of self-esteem and self-assurance. Boundaries help children differentiate between right and wrong, acceptable and unacceptable behavior, and understand the consequences of their actions.

By adhering to established boundaries, children learn to respect themselves and others, establish healthy boundaries in their relationships, and nurture empathy and compassion for others. Boundaries also teach children the importance of personal accountability, integrity, and ethics, which are crucial for character development and earning the trust and respect of others.

The combination of self-discipline and boundaries creates a powerful force, empowering children to become mentally strong, resilient, and self-reliant individuals. Children with self-discipline can set ambitious goals, devise strategies, and take action to pursue their dreams and aspirations. They can overcome obstacles, setbacks, and adversities with unwavering determination and perseverance, strengthening their self-esteem and self-assurance.

Children who are aware of and respect established boundaries can navigate the complexities of social interactions, build healthy and beneficial relationships, and communicate their thoughts and feelings effectively. They can set boundaries that promote their well-being, express their needs and opinions, and assert their rights and beliefs with courage and conviction.

Fostering self-discipline and establishing boundaries are essential for the development and progress of children. These elements not only shape a child's character but also equip them with the skills and values necessary for success and happiness in life. As caregivers and guardians, it is our solemn duty to teach children the importance of self-discipline and boundaries, as it lays the foundation for a future marked by prosperity, harmony, and happiness.

Mental Strength

The true strength of character is developed by confronting adversity with determination. Despite challenges that may test our spirit, an unyielding resilience remains unbroken. It is during our darkest moments that our humanity shines through, not despite hardship, but because of it. Overcoming difficulties allows us to discover our inner strength, moving beyond mere reaction to shape our destiny through proactive willpower. This ability to positively influence our inner world distinguishes mental fortitude as the solid foundation of inner resolve.

At our core, each of us possesses a deep-seated resilience - an innate strength waiting to be cultivated. However, developing mental strength requires intentional effort, as only through conscious strengthening can our inherent resilience reach its full potential. The key question then becomes how to best enhance this latent power within us, turning potential into reality. Building a solid foundation of inner resolve requires understanding the components of fortitude and how they work together. With understanding comes the ability to illuminate the inner workings of strength, giving us the means to enhance it.

Resilience lies at the heart of mental fortitude, forming its sturdy framework. Meaning "to spring back or rebound after compression," resilience involves effectively adapting in the face of adversity or misfortune. Rather than allowing setbacks to discourage or define us, a resilient spirit bounces back from difficulties, maintaining balance and forward momentum even during tough times. Flexibility is critical, as it enables us to weather shocks while retaining our core structure and direction. Those who are resilient possess an elastic nature, bending without breaking under strain as they face challenges with adaptive perseverance.

Closely linked to resilience is perseverance, which provides strength and endurance to fortitude's structure. While resilience allows for adaptation during hardship, perseverance enables sustained effort over the long term. It involves continuing purposeful action despite setbacks, fatigue, or perceived futility. Perseverance draws from a reserve of stamina and tenacity, supplying determined endurance that persists toward goals despite difficulties. Instead of dwelling in frustration, those who persevere stay focused on solutions and progress, adjusting their efforts when plans change and seeing tasks through to completion with unwavering diligence.

Another element that strengthens mental fortitude is an optimistic outlook. Serving as the energizing force behind fortitude, optimism fortifies both resilience and perseverance by influencing perceptions and expectations. An optimist anticipates favorable outcomes, believing that positive results stem more from personal agency than external forces. Even in the face of difficulties, an optimistic perspective focuses on opportunities within challenges and growth potential. An optimistic mindset views challenges through a can-do lens, motivating individuals to weather adversity, find purpose, and discover silver linings where others may only see obstacles. Optimism boosts both energy and the ability to persist through hardships by reframing experiences in a solution-oriented, learning-focused manner.

Closely aligned with optimism, a growth mindset significantly enhances mental fortitude. Unlike a fixed mindset, a growth mindset acknowledges that abilities can be developed through effort over time. Those with a growth mindset believe that personal qualities such as intelligence and talent are malleable, not predetermined limits. They see challenges as opportunities to expand their abilities rather than as proof of inadequacy. A growth mindset fosters resilience by promoting perseverance and instilling the expectation that continued effort can overcome current struggles. It also supports optimism by viewing problems as temporary setbacks in an ongoing developmental journey. A growth mindset broadens the boundaries of what an individual feels they can achieve, giving them greater confidence to overcome adversity and try new approaches.

Self-awareness and self-regulation are key components of mental fortitude. Self-awareness involves understanding one's emotions, thought patterns, strengths, and weaknesses. It leads to self-understanding, fortifies optimism, and enables a more accurate perception of situations. Self-regulation complements self-awareness by providing control over disruptive emotions and impulses through techniques such as stress management, emotion labeling, and cognitive restructuring. The ability to self-regulate strengthens perseverance by channeling energy in a focused, productive direction during difficulties. Mental strength comes from recognizing inner workings and gaining the ability to navigate thoughts, feelings, and behaviors. Thus, awareness and regulation empower fortitude.

Considering these fundamental components reveals how mental fortitude arises through a combination of resilience, perseverance, optimism, a growth mindset, self-awareness, and regulation. While individuals may differ in natural dispositions, life experiences profoundly shape the development of fortitude. Adversity often serves as a crucible in which character strengthens, but how challenges are met makes all the difference. Those with the strongest mental fortitude use difficulties as a way to hone resilience, broaden perspectives, and cultivate persevering determination. By mindfully strengthening the components of fortitude, inherent latent powers are awakened, and abilities are multiplied, establishing a sure foundation of inner resolve capable of weathering any storm.

Throughout history, exemplars of mental fortitude illuminate how cultivated inner strength transforms potential into achievement against all odds. Figures like Nelson Mandela demonstrate the power of fortitude through adverse experiences shaping resilience, perseverance, and leadership. Mandela endured 27 years of imprisonment yet emerged empowered to peacefully dismantle apartheid through reconciliation.

Profiles of courage demonstrate that while external circumstances cannot be controlled, our response to adversity can be shaped. Everyone faces hardships, but our mental strength determines whether we are defeated or grow stronger. Those with strong mental fortitude view challenges as opportunities to expand their skills and wisdom. They use difficulties to become better equipped and more dedicated to their purpose. Adversity acts as a workout for the soul, strengthening our resilience and perseverance as we face each new trial.

Developing mental fortitude helps us positively influence our inner and outer worlds, enabling us to emerge accomplished from life's challenges. Resilience, perseverance, optimism, a growth mindset, self-awareness, and self-regulation work together to form an unbreakable inner foundation. While genetics play a role, our life experiences and daily choices have the greatest impact on developing this determination within us. By consciously strengthening these building blocks - facing setbacks with courage, persistence, and learning - we awaken our inherent powers and transform our potential into actual achievement. True greatness arises from overcoming life's challenges, as mental fortitude refines the human spirit like steel tempered in flame.

A child's most influential teachers shape not only their intellect but also their morals. They mold the humanity within through everyday interactions as well as formal education. As the primary guide for a developing mind, no other relationship has a greater impact on a child's mindset and mental strength. The parental role is both instructive and challenging, carrying significant opportunities and responsibilities. The way parents foster independence while providing security, and embrace mistakes while modeling perseverance, largely determines the character a child develops. Nurturing youth is a great privilege, but it also comes with great accountability as the new generation looks to the older generation for life's most essential lessons.

One of the greatest gifts parents can give to their children is resilience – mental strength developed through overcoming small hardships. Encouraging children to face small failures with reassurance builds their confidence to handle larger challenges in the future. Similar to how a gardener nurtures strong roots by exposing the plant to sun and rain, parents best serve their children by neither over-protecting them nor leaving them to struggle alone, but by walking alongside them and offering guidance. When cultivating character, a balance must be struck between support and self-reliance, nurturing independence by encouraging controlled risk-taking within a safe environment.

Let's consider "helicopter parenting" and its potential negative impacts. Although the intention is to shield children from pain through constant hovering care, the results can undermine the development of independence, which is crucial for resilient adulthood. By removing all obstacles, the toughening trials that build resilience are lost, and dependency replaces confidence. Problems solved prematurely deprive children of the joy of discovery, and completing tasks without struggle diminishes their pride in effort. While kindness may prompt protection, character strengthening arises from facing smaller challenges with loved ones close by, but still requiring independent action. The secure parent-child bond becomes a home base from which children can explore with curiosity, without fear of the natural lessons that come with failure.

Instead of solving all problems, acknowledge and praise the resilient spirit shown in efforts to solve them. Recognize progress even in setbacks to reinforce a growth mindset. Allow natural consequences to occur when safe, such as incomplete tasks resulting in the need for further work, rather than providing instant solutions. Acknowledge and validate emotional responses to small failures, emphasizing them as valuable learning experiences rather than threats to one's worth. This approach allows difficulties to remain challenges that promote independence, rather than problems that require parental intervention, hindering self-reliant progress. Emphasize effort and process over immediate outcomes alone, demonstrating that failures themselves are teachers who assist in achieving success through perseverance.

Model the growth you want to cultivate by demonstrating an attitude that embraces challenges and setbacks. Share your own experiences of building resilience and perseverance through past difficulties, similar to those faced by the child. Show them how resilience comes from within, rather than being dependent on circumstances, and praise their persevering spirit in maintaining a positive mindset through challenges. Encourage them to see that optimism and persistence together build strong resilience.

Where possible, experience failures alongside them, highlighting the benefits that perseverance brings. By facing hardships together, parental leadership can guide youth toward independent problem-solving and bolster their confidence to weather life's inevitable challenges.

Assign responsibilities that match their abilities and provide opportunities for decision-making, while avoiding micromanagement that interferes with autonomy. Respect their privacy boundaries to facilitate identity formation, while remaining approachable for their concerns. Present a united front with co-parents by maintaining consistent standards as children test their limits daily. Acknowledge their efforts and progress, regardless of imperfect results, by celebrating their demonstrated perseverance rather than only rewarding task completion. Allow natural consequences to occur when safe, as independently solving problems sharpens crucial life skills. Guide their progress but avoid over-involvement, striking a balance between nurturing independence and providing safety nets to prevent lasting damage from the difficult lessons of failure.

In a relationship based on respect and trust, taking responsibility leads to ownership and builds intrinsic motivation, gradually replacing the need for external rewards. Show empathy and validate emotions while constructively solving problems to help redirect distress. Be mindful of comparing oneself to others, as it can undermine confidence. Instead, focus on personal growth and improvement over time, rather than comparing to social benchmarks of success. Continuously affirm one's character, which develops regardless of circumstances. Resilient spirits endure challenges through inner strength, not the absence of difficulties. Encourage curiosity, flexibility, and good humor to shape interactions as children develop their identities in a stable home environment, which allows them to venture forth with bravery. Offer unconditional support without manipulation, to strengthen integrity and perseverance through hardships.

Remember that taking care of oneself as a parent is crucial for handling the challenges of raising children. Maintain supportive relationships and engage in rejuvenating activities to reduce stress and prevent exhaustion. Allocate private time for self-care to avoid depletion, which can test your patience and resilience. Striving for perfection as a caregiver is counterproductive; instead, set realistic limits and forgive imperfections to model healthy flexibility and strengthen family bonds. Focus on balancing attending to children's needs with respecting your capacity and needs. Nurturing independence impartially empowers growth, rather than removing adversity, which builds character through trials. Embrace flexibility to meet the evolving developmental changes with understanding.

Above all, prioritize cultivating secure child-caregiver bonds, as they form the most influential attachment in life. Resilience flourishes when there is unconditional regard and acceptance despite imperfections. This secure attachment fosters the confidence to explore independence, knowing there is a stable home base to return to. Confidence in facing adversity comes from the experience of retaining self-worth despite circumstances, shaped by a nurturing environment that models empathy, understanding, and perseverance in partnership. Such compassion sustains motivation through setbacks, as difficulties both strengthen character and reveal internal fortitude, which requires safety to emerge undaunted.

Through guidance empowering autonomy and mutual care sustaining security, parents shape the conditions for children to develop life's most protective quality: an inner resilience reinforced by independent victories large and small. By welcoming small storms as opportunities rather than problems, resilience's protective muscle strengthens for facing greater forces of change ahead. Through parental leadership empowering self-guided progress, character emerges fortified to weather challenges independently yet supported by family bonds of unconditional care. Such secure foundations nurture humanity with the potential to impact lives positively across generations – as any seed requiring sun and rain takes root, so too under wise encouragement does resilience spread its sheltering branches for all who follow to find shade.

Life's journey proves unpredictable, with unknown terrain certain to harbor hidden obstacles and opportunities alike. To weather inevitable difficulties - whether imposed from without or arising within - requires an inner strength flexible yet durable, adaptable yet steady. This power of resilience enables turning even hardships to advantage, emerging empowered rather than defeated by circumstance. Though outer events prove beyond personal control, the mind's response can be cultivated through focused intention. Resilience arises from within as a matter of habit and perspective, bolstered through daily choices nurturing emotional intelligence alongside persevering spirit. By consciously strengthening fortitude's sources, inherent potential blossoms into assured fulfillment when facing any storm.

At resilience's heart lies flexibility - an ability to bend without breaking under life's shifting pressures. Flexibility demands acknowledging present limitations and environmental constraints without surrendering agency or abandoning growth. It preserves progress and principled purpose through change by widening perspective beyond immediate conditions. Flexible spirits roll with life's punches by reframing difficulties as temporary yet instructive, focusing effort where influence remains while accepting realities beyond direct impact. This detached yet engaged outlook sustains progress amid obstacles through prudent adaptation guided by a higher purpose.

Allied with flexibility is perseverance - the unwavering will that enables continued effort despite setbacks or perceived futility. Perseverance draws from reserves of patience, dedication, and tenacity, allowing individuals to carry on constructively toward valued goals despite difficulties. Instead of becoming frustrated, perseverance maintains focus on realistic solutions and incremental wins, forming foundations for future growth. It channels efforts productively when plans need revision, seeing tasks through to reasoned completion with diligent persistence. Perseverance strengthens resilience by refusing to yield where principles remain intact and improvement is still possible through a proactive will.

Closely related, emotional intelligence enhances resilience through self-awareness, self-regulation, and social adroitness. Self-awareness involves deeply understanding one's thought patterns, emotions, and tendencies. It helps build realistic perspectives on strengths and limits, enabling the assessment of challenges within one's capacities. Self-regulation allows individuals to channel responses constructively through techniques like labeling feelings, cognitive reframing, and stress management. Emotional intelligence also encompasses empathy, social conscientiousness, and conflict navigation - interpersonal skills that fortify connections and sustain purpose and well-being through difficulties. Together, awareness and mastery of emotions bolster persevering through life's changes.

Optimism serves as a wellspring of continued effort, seeing difficulties as temporary and growth as possible. It perceives setbacks through a solution-focused lens, believing that effort and creative thinking can overcome hardships through persevering spirit and openness to alternatives. Instead of dwelling on the problem, optimism concentrates on opportunities within the challenge and potential lessons that further understanding and wisdom. It sustains perseverance through hard times by reframing circumstances upliftingly as passing yet instructive phases of an overall developmental journey. Optimism means "seeing the good," maintaining an encouraging outlook that empowers flexible adaptation.

Cultivating gratitude also nurtures fortitude. Adopting an attitude appreciative of life's simple gifts sparks joy amid deeper trials. Gratitude recognizes goodness amid imperfection, focusing on abundance and blessings present rather than wanting for more. It enables maintaining perspective through difficulties by redirecting attention to fundamentals sustaining well-being. Expressing gratitude through journaling, prayers, and sharing strengthens social bonds, bolstering perseverance. Combined, optimism and gratitude form resilient spirits' nourishing daily regimen, sustaining will and flexibility through challenges by reframing problems as passing phases within fortunate contexts.

A growth mindset empowers meeting obstacles encouragingly, believing capabilities emerge and evolve in response to effort rather than limitation. Growth orientation perceives setbacks as opportunities to expand understanding and skill rather than intrinsic defects. It sustains perseverance by expecting continued learning through difficulties and viewing adversity as temporary versus defining. A growth perspective understands humans as works constantly in progress, naturally developing capabilities proportional to endeavor across lifetimes, enabling challenge-embracing attitudes bolstering flexible adaptation. Together, optimism, gratitude, and a growth mindset nurture resilient fortitude, sustaining spirituality.

Additional practices cultivating resilience include savoring life's smaller pleasures through mindfulness, expressing emotions constructively via creativity, practicing good humor, prioritizing rest, and maintaining supportive social circles. Together with patience and diligent effort, these daily choices progressively strengthen fortitude's reliable reserves accessed through changing tides. Resilience emerges through conscious renewal nourishing persevering spirit amid inevitable tests of endurance, an inherent human capacity awakened through grit, gratitude, and gladness daily reinforced.

In developing inner strength, renew your perseverance each day through practicing gratitude, compassion, and embracing possibility. Human resilience thrives when we consciously nurture it and build a strong yet flexible character. With this approach, we can overcome any challenge and emerge stronger, and more committed to self-improvement. While difficulties may arise unexpectedly, fortitude is a result of focused intention and daily choices. May everyone find the strength to persevere through challenges and changes, unlocking the gifts of resilience within themselves.

The challenges of modern life are constantly changing, but the basic needs of human beings remain the same. While technology is advancing rapidly and connecting us globally, our psychological makeup stays consistent. To help young people grow into resilient and principled individuals who can navigate life's uncertainties, we need to instill certain core virtues from an early age.

Understanding mental strength, which includes resilience, perseverance, and optimism, can help us cope with inevitable challenges. Having a growth mindset, where we see challenges as opportunities to learn and grow, can help us develop this strength. Self-awareness and self-regulation also help us thoughtfully handle difficult situations.

The family unit plays a crucial role in shaping a child's psychological development. A parent's behavior and attitude have a profound impact on their child's growth. While it's natural for parents to want to protect and care for their children, being overly controlling can hinder a child's ability to become independent and solve problems on their own. It's important to guide without being overbearing, allowing children to make mistakes and learn from them, which helps them develop resilience. Leading by example, showing composure during tough times, and celebrating small victories can help instill these qualities. Building trust and fostering open communication can also help nurture inner strength.

Resilience, the ability to persevere through tough times, is closely tied to emotional intelligence. Being aware of one's emotions, exercising self-control, and being able to empathize with others all contribute to developing resilience. Practices such as gratitude, viewing challenges as opportunities for growth, and developing various coping mechanisms can help strengthen one's ability to weather life's challenges. Stories of individuals who have overcome great adversity through resilience serve as a reminder that our greatest strengths often emerge during difficult times.

Self-respect and confidence come from within but are influenced by external factors. When parents emphasize effort over innate talent, praise the learning process rather than just the results, and avoid excessive praise or criticism, children can develop a strong sense of self-esteem grounded in virtues rather than fleeting emotions. This approach helps children see themselves as works in progress, constantly improving and problem-solving. Instilling a deep sense of each child's inherent worth and potential for positive change helps build a wellspring of inner confidence.

While there's no foolproof way to shield children from life's challenges, focusing on nurturing their psychological strength, balanced perspective, emotional mastery, and a strong sense of purpose and self-worth can provide them with the tools to thrive. Fostering strong character in our children is a profound and enduring responsibility and our most noble legacy. With compassion and wisdom, let's rise to the challenge for the benefit of future generations.

Leading by Example

The influence of parents on a child's development is profound. Children learn essential life lessons by observing their parents' everyday actions, rather than through explicit teaching. As children seek to understand the world and their place in it, they naturally internalize the behaviors they see regularly. Therefore, the role of parents is invaluable and carries significant responsibility in shaping a child's character.

Research consistently shows that parental actions strongly predict children's outcomes. A supportive home environment predicts positive attributes such as confidence, strong relationships, and academic success. Children not only internalize abstract principles but also observe and learn from the integrity and moral habits of their parents. The influence of parental behavior is more significant than mere words, as children learn from the patterns they see habitually rewarded or discouraged around them.

Communication styles within the family also play a crucial role in a child's development. Constructive discussions model emotional regulation, empathy, and principled resolution. Patient and firm responses to frustrations teach children appropriate ways to manage their frustrations. On the other hand, harsh, unpredictable, or insincere interactions can predict later relationship issues for children. Parents' respectful and open communication styles help children feel secure in exploring and expressing themselves, fostering independence balanced with responsibility.

Parents not only guide what children learn but also influence how they process information and relate to others. Their conduct shapes children's social-emotional development more than direct education.

When it comes to discipline, consistently enforcing fair consequences helps children learn self-control. Explaining the reasons behind rules helps children understand and accept them, leading to cooperation instead of rebellion. Reward systems encourage positive behavior, such as praising perseverance instead of just avoiding misbehavior. Discipline, when used wisely, becomes an opportunity to teach children self-restraint and independence, which are important for their development. Being too permissive can lead to spoiling while being too harsh can stem from caregivers' unmet needs. It's important to balance structure with warmth and to maintain authority with calmness and respect to preserve family bonds.

The development of a strong work ethic comes from observing consistent efforts and facing challenges with dignity. This instills a reward for perseverance in the face of adversity, rather than expecting entitlement over temporary setbacks. Parents teach diligence by demonstrating the importance of sticking to schedules, honoring commitments despite challenges, and calmly completing responsibilities fully and on time. By dedicating themselves to mutual improvement through honest self-improvement, they set an example of gradual progress through daily small improvements, rather than expecting overnight change. Self-sacrifice for the sake of loved ones teaches gratitude, compassion, and the value of serving the community. On the other hand, procrastination, dishonesty, or blaming others can lead to modeling irresponsibility, whereas integrity strengthens relationships and promotes fair cooperation.

Being a role model requires daily self-reflection, adaptation, and a willingness to demonstrate lifelong learning. Admitting imperfections and areas for growth with humility maintains credibility, as it shows that nobody is perfect, but progress comes through effort and shared experiences. Showing forgiveness towards others and oneself builds resilience against making surface-level judgments. Prioritizing relationships over materialism can prevent discontentment despite inevitable challenges. Creating an environment of calmness, playfulness, and gratitude nourishes empathy, rather than causing stress that harms essential bonds for overall wellness. Balancing indulgence and strictness teaches moderation, supporting autonomy within reason. Ultimately, maintaining overall health, involvement, and fulfillment signifies life's deeper rewards through responsible stewardship.

Parenting guidance is an ongoing task that requires mindful guardians to lead with integrity, setting examples that gradually shape the character of their children. Each generation is influenced by the previous one, so few duties carry as much importance as parenting well. All guardians need to embrace the privilege with humility and care, as they are entrusted with the development of their children. By cultivating integrity, compassion, and diligence from an early age, a foundation is laid for establishing justice, community, and truth. These humble yet significant tasks give everyday interactions ultimate significance, as the slow blossoming of character unfolds from examples witnessed in the home.

Compassion, kindness, and empathy are innate in every soul, but they require moral cultivation and nurturing to flourish. These virtues form the fertile soil from which just, peaceful, and fulfilled societies naturally grow. They are habits that are intentionally cultivated through mindful living, learned behaviors that emerge gradually through principled examples, relationships, and experiences over time. Each small act has consequences that ripple outward, affecting unknown shores. Therefore, daily conduct holds profound yet subtle power to nourish humanity or leave it wanting. With privilege comes the duty to foster compassion, so that shared benevolence may multiply where seeds fall.

Kindness is the act of showing thoughtful care towards all people and creatures while respecting their inherent dignity and differences. It involves understanding and addressing conflict and improving conditions for others through voluntary aid. Kindness bridges social rifts and fosters goodwill, without expecting anything in return. It recognizes the basic decency of all individuals and counteracts prejudices through outward-focused compassion. Small gestures like smiles, favors, and compliments can cultivate empathy and uplift communities. Respect, on the other hand, acknowledges each individual's autonomy and right to their own experiences. It respects privacy, avoids judgment, and affirms personal agency while seeking collaborative resolutions. Respect appreciates diversity of thought and appearance, finding value in varied perspectives. Open dialogue and patience help to maintain integrity and foster shared understanding, even amid disagreement. Through respect, shared understanding can emerge where division once reigned, as all sides are considered respectfully.

Empathy completes the triad of compassion by imagining experiences from a different perspective and sympathizing with a range of emotions. It helps us understand how behaviors affect different members of society and holds justice and mercy in a balanced regard. Empathy softens initial reactions by encouraging thoughtful perspective-taking and promotes communal betterment by addressing issues without judgment. It fosters fellowship in adversity and avoids "othering" by appealing to our common humanity. Empathy humanizes all parties in conflicts by recognizing shared vulnerabilities with kindness and understanding. Kindness, respect, and empathy together build community bonds that uplift everyone.

Cultivating compassion requires consistent, small efforts, as virtuous habits are formed gradually through daily living. It involves practicing courtesy, listening without judgment, helping those in need, and alleviating suffering wherever possible. Forgiving imperfections in oneself and others, avoiding harsh language, respecting opposing beliefs, and finding shared interests are all ways to unite differences. Expressing gratitude frequently through words and actions reminds us of life's simple gifts and shifts our perspectives outwardly. Voluntary community participation through collectively practiced virtues magnifies their impact, as kindness multiplies through shared actions.

Education instills these habits early by modeling respect, cultivating curious yet empathetic minds, and fostering the dignity of all peoples through accurate historical representation. The media also holds responsibility by avoiding sensationalism that degrades the common good, and instead highlighting shared hopes and virtues commendably. Leaders who rally cooperation through equitable policies, rather than divisiveness, nourish justice and prosperity for all. Overall, a shared civic spirit upholds virtues like fairness, and strengthening social bonds in practice rather than precept alone. Together, small steps sustain compassion, and flowering where sown through daily renewals of character.

Challenges may arise, but virtue persists through principled perseverance. Considerate communication can resolve conflicts respectfully. Even in inevitable disagreements, integrity should be reflected in the manner expressed rather than in position alone. Compassion can counter hardening tendencies through forgiveness and seeking resolution over retribution. Adversity presents an opportunity to strengthen fortitude through proactivity, creativity, and keeping vision fixed on shared hopes rather than momentary limitations. Overall moderation, balance, and humility should guide conduct amid complexity and uncertainty.

By practicing mindfulness and maintaining a persevering spirit, daily compassion can become a habit. Let's all reflect on cultivating kindness, respect, and empathy so that our communities may thrive in understanding where once there were divisions. By uplifting one another through consideration of our shared hopes, shared prosperity naturally follows, much like overflowing waters nourish the fertile plains below.

Existence brings uncertainties that will inevitably lead to difficulties, as external stresses intersect with humanity's inner struggles. How individuals handle life's challenges depends on their focus and moderately applied willpower. Difficult situations test one's character, revealing strength and resilience through maintaining integrity and humanity despite tough conditions. Grace represents virtuous strength that guides us through turbulence by focusing on principles, even when everything else seems to be falling apart. Adversity presents opportunities to strengthen our spirit or weaken under pressure; maintaining composure allows us to face trials while upholding dignity for ourselves and others through unwavering calm.

Developing principled composure requires cultivating emotional intelligence, and recognizing our inner landscape and tendencies through self-reflection. Self-awareness acknowledges our subjective biases and habitual reactions, allowing us to steer our emotions willfully by focusing on the fundamentals. Identifying triggers prepares us to navigate difficulties intentionally, despite our vulnerabilities. Sustaining self-awareness through honest improvement nurtures integrity when facing external stresses.

Self-regulation strategies help to channel reactions constructively. By naming feelings dispassionately, intensity is defused, allowing for a choice in response. Deep breathing releases tension, while a clarified perspective redirects towards resolution. Affirming core convictions helps to maintain direction. Redirecting distressed thoughts refocuses outward through empathy and community. Together, awareness and willpower maintain integrity as an anchor amid disarray.

Empathy strengthens resilience by imagining others' experiences with compassion. Perspective expands beyond self-interest to the community's well-being, acting as a shared vessel weathering storms. Empathy resolves conflicts by respecting all parties' humanity despite maintained disagreements. It humanizes "opponents" by envisioning shared hopes beneath behaviors, enabling reconciliations where convictions are preserved. Together, awareness, regulation, and empathy navigate turbulence, upholding dignity for self and others through principled fortitude.

Adversity arises, but virtues remain through moderation. Consider the drivers of tension and respond proportionately yet resolutely. Address underlying issues constructively while avoiding escalations that worsen situations. Communicate calmly and actively listen to others' perspectives, even if they were initially unheard. Find collaborative solutions that uplift all sides' integrity, avoiding retribution or forcing compliance that disrespects autonomy. Approach interactions as opportunities to strengthen relationships wherever resolution remains possible.

Resilience is strengthened through reframing hardships optimistically. Regard difficulties as passing chapters of learning rather than defeats of worth. Focus on progress made and lessons learned, broadening understanding. Maintain hopeful attributions, interpreting setbacks as temporary yet instructive experiences within overall growth. Persevere challenges by channeling effort resourcefully despite impediments. Optimize circumstances within our influence rather than fixating on limitations. With patience and flexibility, resilience carries resolutions forward through life's shifting complexities.

Composure arises through facing each adversity as a chance to prove virtue's measure. By centering on principles, navigating turbulence maintains integrity and humanity despite outward disorder. Grace signifies strength guiding conduct rightly amid disruption. With practice, composure becomes a resilient habit, weathering life's unpredictabilities through steady focus, and upholding self and community. May all face trials of endurance, sustaining spirit and dignity through regulating responses proportionately yet principled. In withstanding difficulties gracefully emerges the character's surest mettle - carrying resolutions forward with poised fortitude.

The rearing of psychologically vigorous youth stands as a monumental responsibility for any conscientious guardian. While external forces like technological advancement and societal evolution continually rework the landscape of modern living, fostering strength of character remains the surest preparation for both calamity and opportunity. Through compassionate guidance and lifelong modeling of integrity, parents sculpt the inner architecture upon which children build their understanding of self and relations with others.

Positive leadership, achieved through open communication, fair discipline, and displaying virtuous behavior, helps individuals thrive. On the other hand, exposure to negativity can cause inner turmoil and hinder healthy development. Leading with patience, empathy, and trust encourages open and honest conversations, allowing for correction without suppressing individuality or spirit. Discipline without scorn fosters responsibility instead of resentment.

Modeling kindness, respect, and compassion promotes harmony within homes and communities, emphasizing our shared humanity. Regular practice of these qualities strengthens virtuous behavior as a natural habit. Kindness brings warmth and uplifts others, respect acknowledges the dignity of all people, and empathy fosters understanding beyond one's own experiences. Educating future generations about these virtues equips them to combat indifference, with the family serving as the most solid foundation.

Life inevitably presents challenges. Adversity can strike without warning. During these difficult times, staying composed and responding gracefully shows strong character. Reacting with anger and distress only leads to more negativity. Keeping a clear mind allows for thoughtful responses and the chance for reconciliation. Remaining calm under pressure prevents impulsive reactions and sets a positive example for others. Inner peace and determination help navigate through turbulent times. Developing resilience through mindfulness, self-awareness, and healthy perspectives prepares us for when difficulties arise.

By consistently embodying these virtues, our home becomes a fortress of character, and our children learn valuable lessons. They understand that challenges build strength and wisdom through reflection. They learn that differences can be handled with care and that showing consideration and compassion lights the way in dark times. Instilling this depth of spirit and strength prepares our children to not just endure life's complexities, but to actively engage and contribute. It teaches them to approach each day with integrity, wonder, service, and kindness despite uncertainties.

Passing on these lessons creates a chain of conscientious guardians and offers hope for society.

While demonstrating strength, parents must avoid replicating the flaws of being inflexible. Wisdom acknowledges life's rich ambiguities. With understanding and nuance, the righteous path forward emerges through open-mindedness, not obstinacy alone. By focusing on cultivating noble character, balanced perspective, and grace within children, we nurture roots from which resilience, compassion, and purpose may forever flourish throughout life's seasons. This stands among a parent's highest callings. If embraced with diligence, our efforts ripple outward, leaving future generations better equipped to weather

any adversity – and empowered to uplift all of
humanity.

Communication

Among a home's most vital bonds stands communication—the exchange of ideas, feelings, and experiences that build understanding between loved ones. Relationships serve as vessels conveying humanity's passage through life's journeys. As voyagers share trials, joys, and visions while supporting one another's burdens, connections deepen most profoundly through shared fellowship. Communication doesn't happen by chance but requires intentional nurturing—mindful cultivation that demands focus yet yields rewards compounding over time. By exchanging openly yet caringly, harmony finds root where potential disunion may have existed, and through enriching each other's lives, families become sanctuaries nourishing the soul.

Effective communication cultivates understanding through active engagement, prioritizing clarity, and respecting various perspectives. Misunderstandings arise from withheld intents or impressions; honesty gently shared relieves unnecessary tensions. Making time for face-to-face communication honors relationships as replenishing wells from which all may drink. Technology's conveniences complement but cannot replace in-person communion. Calm discussion resolves issues cooperatively, addressing root concerns with dignity while maintaining the integrity of spirit.

Shared fellowship nourishes empathy through perspective. By envisioning life through another's experiences, compassion grows where detachment may have existed. Differences enlighten when appreciated, not merely tolerated, as diverse arrays teach more than uniform solitudes. Active listening focuses full presence on the speaker, reflecting their essence to confirm understanding of intentions as they were meant, avoiding projections. Silences show care for words' weight rather than fleeing discomfort.

Compassion should guide our speech, uplifting everyone through our interactions. If criticism is necessary, it should be delivered lovingly, while affirming the inherent goodness in each person, despite their flaws. Gratitude should remind us of the gifts we have received, and forgiveness should come easily, as we all have our imperfections and shared vulnerabilities. Anger serves no purpose, so we should strive for calmness, allowing resolutions to emerge gradually through patience as storms subside.

Setting intentions helps to bring people closer, creating space in our busy lives for meaningful connections beyond just sharing information. Engaging in shared activities provides an opportunity to truly get to know one another without distractions. Asking gentle questions about well-being and dreams, without judgment, validates both struggles and triumphs, however, they are expressed. Physical touch, hugs, and maintaining eye contact convey presence where words may fail. Comfortable silences signify peace between companions, showing closeness through being present for one another.

It's important to recognize that different generations have different needs and capacities, and we should adjust to maintain connectedness. Respecting boundaries as lives expand is crucial, especially for teens who need autonomy alongside guidance. Compromise allows for graceful accommodation of change while addressing conflict constructively leads to growth. Preserving fleeting "peace" through stifled discourse comes at the cost of true understanding, whereas forgiveness and second chances can rebuild what strictness may destroy.

Overall communication cultivates community within the home, where fellowship nourishes the soul. By embracing shared lives as a blessing deserving mindful nurturance, understanding deepens steadily through laughter and tears together. May all dwell in compassionate relation, uplifting one another through calm yet honest interaction, so that mutual care may spread its branches, sheltering all who find rest in each other's company through life's mingled sorrows and delights.

For emotions prove universal yet variably expressed; and while natural reactions arise transiently, capabilities develop gradually through guidance, empowering healthy expression. Yet navigating feelings requires tools beyond inborn tendencies, necessitating intentional nurturance empowering emotional regulation, self-awareness, and empathy essential for well-being. Here, a parent proves to be an invaluable mentor, whose support cultivates durable inner resources enabling composure despite life's complexities. With privilege comes the duty to nourish emotional intelligence from seeds within, so that character may blossom resiliently.

Discussing feelings teaches identification and vocabulary and permits one to experience a full range naturally. This validates emotions rather than repressing or over-intellectualizing reactions. Brief check-ins help name often fleeting sentiments and perspectives that form understanding. Asking open-ended questions shows active care for inner experiences however expressed. Mirroring back what's heard confirms comprehension of another's interior landscape, avoiding assumptions through empathetic reflection.

Modeling vulnerability through calm sharing of one's feelings permits children to openly feel however they do. This conveys emotions as natural rather than weaknesses, strengthening trust that feelings won't be met with alarm or derision whatever their nature. Parents guide by example that feelings simply are - warranting neither judgment nor action alone but thoughtful navigation. Discussing constructive strategies for various emotions provides tools amid inevitable difficulties.

Consider children's developmental capacities in discussions. Toddlers can learn to identify basic emotions through books, games, or creative artwork that explores feelings. With guidance, school-agers can discuss triggers, causes, and effects. Teens appreciate perspective-taking on complex experiences and advice that respects their autonomy. Gentle, age-appropriate discussions can help nurture emotional intelligence adaptively across childhood.

Encourage various safe outlets for expressing emotions. Creative exercises such as drawing, music, dance, or journaling can help release inner experiences. Physical activities can channel the energy produced by strong feelings productively. Spending time in nature can help alleviate distress. Constructive problem-solving can address underlying issues and reduce negative emotions. Venting judiciously can help maintain perspective, reminding us that feelings are simply experiences to navigate thoughtfully, not identities to wallow in or stifle.

Avoid minimizing or dismissing feelings, as this can inhibit expression and regulation. Validate another person's inner state through calm reflection, even if it's unpleasant, to avoid invalidation that might lead to withdrawn communication. Affirm that everyone sometimes feels similarly and encourage finding healthy ways of responding thoughtfully. Discuss alternative strategies to harmful outlets like self-harm, outbursts, or vices. Optimize the situation where safe, without fixating unhelpfully on difficulties alone, and maintain hope that feelings naturally ebb and flow within happier contexts.

Self-care and community support can bolster resilience when navigating difficult emotions. Prioritize rest, nutrition, fresh air, and recreation to support mental wellness. Spending time in nature can alleviate stress through the perspective-broadening effects of awe. Maintaining close relationships allows both giving and receiving comfort through shared experiences, even when it's individually difficult. Overall balance can prevent harmful fixations on demanding external or internal forces.

With gentle yet patient guidance, emotional intelligence grows steadily from nurturing inner experiences openly yet constructively. May all cultivate this invaluable life skill empowering fulfillment despite difficulties inevitable. By cultivating awareness, empathy, and healthy regulation of feelings from within, character emerges resiliently navigating complexities with poised fortitude and grace.

An often overlooked but profoundly impactful aspect of the care lies in cultivating empathy - the ability to walk in another's shoes by perceiving experiences from their point of view. Empathy strengthens bonds of trust that lay the foundations for cooperation, competence, and resilience as our little ones navigate life's complexities. Yet developing this sensitivity requires attentiveness and example on our part, so that young minds may practice perceiving beyond superficial actions into deeper essence. With patience and compassion, we guide our youth toward perceiving life's diversity as sources of shared fellowship rather than division alone.

Active listening forms the doorway to empathy, necessitating full presence with our children free from distraction or projections. Making eye contact, facing them fully yet non-threateningly, and occasional verbal and physical responses signal openness to understand another's inner experience. Reflecting in our own words what we gather they mean to convey without assumptions confirms comprehension of their intended message. Clarifying questions seek to accurately sense personal sights, sounds, feelings, and needs as described, avoiding injecting our narrative. Pausing thoughtfully before responding keeps the focus on the speaker instead of fleeting to advise or debate prematurely.

Listening with the intent to truly hear another's essence models the valuation of each perspective however novel to our own. It teaches that diverse viewpoints need not conflict but broaden shared awareness when appreciated integrally. Validating another's humanity and intrinsic worth emerges through perceptions sensitively received without censorship or hasty conclusions. Children feel affirmed that they and others matter, seeding empathy from security that one will be openly heard and understood in return whenever needs arise. Our patience and presence consoling tender minds grant permission to share fears or failures confident support rather than alienation awaits.

Once actively empathized, perspective expands to envision scenarios from another's vantage point - be they family, community member, or beyond. Imaginatively considering life through another's eyes, feelings, culture or conditions cultivates compassion for a diversity of journeys. Appreciating varied yet shared human experiences naturally breeds fellowship over divisions superficially perceived. Empathy sensitizes to impacts of behaviors and speech beyond self-focused intentions, nurturing conscientious growth attuned to communities reliant on mutual care. By opening awareness to life's rich multiplicities experienced variously yet unitedly, empathy nourishes spiritual depth perceiving life's interwoven fabric.

Validating emotions conveyed and acknowledging situations imagined from an alternative vantage model of emotional empathy. Verbalizing an understanding of another's feelings without judgment teaches that all emotions simply are - warranting navigable experiences that link humans despite superficial contrasts. Dismissing no one's inner reality preserves dignity for varied expressions however dissimilar initially to our own. Compassion holds space for discomfort non-threateningly, acknowledging shared hopes beneath transient sentiments and keeping relationships intact through disagreements. Our words and manner nurture confidence that empathy shall listen without punitive reactions whatever arises.

In practicing these attentive skills ourselves, we guide our little ones' earliest encounters with diversity - be it in ability, appearance, background, or belief. From infancy, our interactions with seed sensitivities take root through daily growth. May our parenthood cultivate this invaluable quality strengthening character with care, insight, and benevolence, so that our youth emerge attuned to life's interconnections empowering justice, cooperation, and shalom wherever footsteps fall. By nurturing empathy, we nourish the ideals of an open-hearted community - empowering coming generations to meet an intricately entwined world with humility, generosity, and grace.

Effective communication requires diligent cultivation. By consciously setting aside time for thoughtful discussion, barriers to openness can be dismantled. Active listening through focused eye contact and reflection indicates valued presence. Empathizing without judgment invites vulnerability. Communication thus becomes a conduit, not just for exchanging facts but for conveying care, respect, and trust through attentiveness to each other's experiences.

Crucial to communication is teaching children to identify and articulate inner experiences. Recognition and labeling of emotions regulate the physiological turmoil that arises during distressing moments. It enhances self-awareness which bolsters resilience when navigating life's uncertainties. By supporting careful expression of feelings through emotional validation, children learn emotions need not overwhelm but can be safely processed. They come to see challenges as opportunities to strengthen interconnectivity within the family unit rather than threats to stability.

Cultivating empathy allows walking in another's shoes, if but for a moment. Through active listening - suspending one's preconceptions to genuinely hear another - families foster profound interconnectedness. It conveys that each member's inner life deserves comprehension and compassion. Minor and large hurts alike find balm through empathetic reflection. Children see themselves as valued individuals whose feelings matter, breeding self-assuredness and consideration for others.

Of course, as with any complex process, setbacks will occur. Misunderstandings are inevitable amid humanity's frailties and life's uncertainties. However, by consciously prioritizing compassionate dialogue through diverse means - expressing care, listening without judgment, and reflecting on another's experience - the bonds of understanding and trust deepen inexorably. Families become sanctuaries where each member's intrinsic worth is affirmed through mutual regard. Children learn relationships thrive not from conflict avoidance, but from facing difficulties with patience, empathy, and good faith.

These interpersonal strengths, when internalized from an early age, become life tools honed through practice. Children absorb that authentic connection arises from honesty, not superficial harmony alone. They grasp challenges need not divide if approached with nuance, care for others' perspectives, and belief in reconciliation. Equipped thus, they engage the world with psychological depth and humility, rather than fear or hostility towards life's ambiguities. In turn, pass on these relationship virtues as stewards of the community.

Of course, perfection is beyond any household. But by consistently making a conscious effort to foster open, empathetic communication as a priority, families optimize conditions for members to weather inevitable stresses. Children learn relationships require cultivation, not demand, and that sharing life's burdens through understanding and support breeds resilience within and between all people. This stands as a parent's most profound teaching and enduring gift to future generations.

Clear Boundaries

One of the most crucial responsibilities of a parent is to foster a child's healthy growth and development by offering intentional guidance. When children are born, they are reliant on others and lack an inherent comprehension of intricate social norms and potential dangers that need to be navigated. During these critical early years, it is imperative to set clear boundaries that provide a sense of security, allowing children to explore their independence within a safe environment. Boundaries should not be seen solely as restrictions, but as valuable tools that teach important life skills such as self-control, empathy, and accountability, which are crucial for building character. It is a significant privilege for parents to lay the foundation for their children to navigate the world thoughtfully and constructively.

A boundary signifies a perceived border demarcating what is and is not acceptable regarding one's physical body, emotions, behaviors, time, or possessions. Healthy boundaries prevent confusion over another's agency while respecting one's own. Several boundary types require consideration for balanced development. Physical boundaries protect bodily autonomy through appropriate physical contact and space. Emotional boundaries involve processing experiences and connecting with others in constructive ways respecting all parties' comfort. Behavioral boundaries regulate courteous conduct toward self and others. Temporal and ownership boundaries give structure allowing focus and ownership over choices.

From infancy, children learn boundaries through parents' consistent, caring responses establishing predictable expectations. By respecting a baby's physical and emotional cues, parents gently teach consent and agency over their gradually developing self. Touch requires permission signaled nonverbally at first, teaching bodily autonomy. Timely responses to cries prevent distress teaching needs eliciting care. Over time, verbal and physical affection requires reciprocal willingness, as understanding grows. These foundations empower navigating intimacy appropriately, meeting discomfort calmly while validating the experience.

As mobility and independence increase, boundaries necessitate expansion appropriately matched to comprehension. Direct supervision gives way to open yet watchful observation, as physical boundaries relax and more nuanced social expectations emerge. Children begin comprehending ownership, schedules, and shared space constraints through structuring daily routines and clarifying varied locations' purposes (playroom vs. kitchen, for example). Natural consequences expedite understanding limits' impacts, like put-away toys before playing with others teaching priorities.

Guidance sustains coherence by explaining changes to boundaries rationally and consistently enforcing reasonable consequences. Physical punishment proves counterproductive, fostering resentment and rebellion instead of intrinsic compliance. However, logical links between behaviors and results redirect children helpfully. Praise cooperation and independence emerging within safeguards, not defiance requiring intervention. Overall, boundaries empower rather than confine when imparted through empathy, patience, and reason rather than reaction.

Teaching safety necessitates addressing the real risks children face. Discussing private areas, secrets, consent, and bodily autonomy gives vocabulary empowering disclosure of discomfort. Explain inappropriate contacts clearly without inducing fear, counterbalanced by openness building trusting relationships children feel safe within. Internet safety, stranger danger, and hazards complement life skills like phone numbers, addresses, problem-solving, and help-seeking cultivated incrementally with independence. Overall, safety emerges from empowered understanding rather than ignorance regarding changing capacities.

Boundaries define behaviors respecting self and others, and imparting social and emotional intelligence. Children glean appropriate conduct subtly through exposure rather than overt instruction alone. Considerate interactions model empathy, compromise, and regulating responses constructively. Guidance addresses hurting feelings calmly while validating perspectives and encouraging cooperation. Conflict resolution skills enable peaceful solutions respecting all. Praise efforts and progress, not perfection alone, cultivating resilience and meeting challenges with perseverance.

Structure provides security enabling safe independence manifested through instilling inner discipline progressively replacing external controls. Reasonable chores build responsibility alongside competencies. Choices foster autonomy within sensible parameters respecting others. Overall, boundaries empower through establishing limitations enabling youth to positively engage life's unpredictabilities from a place of provision and trust. May all who guide developing lives embrace this privilege with sage care, imparting stability and self-regulation nurturing character from within.

Guiding children toward cultivating integrity, wisdom, and virtue is a formidable task that requires diligence, empathy, and discernment. Parents play an integral role in assisting young ones to comprehend the distinction between behaviors that uplift and those that degrade. Fostering this discernment entails communicating expectations while allowing room for mistakes from which valuable lessons can be learned. Through compassionate yet consistent direction, little ones gain the ability to independently navigate complexity and make choices befitting their inherent nobility.

Establishing a framework of principles is crucial for helping children understand what constitutes respectful conduct. Principles emerge from deep introspection on elevating human dignity and relationships. They help children recognize how certain acts diminish personal worth or harm others. Some key principles include respect, compassion, honesty, and responsibility. Explaining why these virtues matter cultivates wisdom. For instance, respect acknowledges the inherent value in all people so we avoid hurtful speech or violating boundaries. Compassion means considering how one's actions impact others to prevent causing distress.

Instilling principles requires ongoing guidance tailored to a child's comprehension. Relating lessons to their world through stories, activities, and open discussion aids retention. Principles also evolve as children mature. Maintaining respectful dialog allows revisiting ideas to explore new depths of meaning. While discipline corrects lapses, the aim is not punishment but growth in character. With patience and understanding, little ones internalize principles as a lens for navigating choices during their journey of self-discovery.

Once anchored in principles, children can grasp nuanced expectations for specific settings and situations. Examples clarify appropriate conduct in areas like family interactions, school, friendships, and extracurricular activities. Positive expectations reinforce conduct upholding dignity rather than those hindering it. For instance:

At home, be respectful of others by not interrupting, using manners, and cooperating with chores.

In school, focus on learning through active listening, participating helpfully, and completing assignments.

With peers, demonstrating kindness, sharing, taking turns, and resolving conflicts respectfully.

During activities, giving full effort, good sportsmanship and not endangering safety.

Unacceptable opposite behaviors are identified, like aggression, damage to property, or academic dishonesty. Consequences for these are reviewed respectfully without harshness to encourage better choices. Illustrating the thoughtfulness behind standards empowers children to comprehend their role in contributing positively. With guidance, they grasp conduct facilitating well-being versus what infringes on it.

For children to internalize expectations, consistency in enforcement is paramount. This involves fairly applying the same outcomes each time standards are not met. Inconsistency breeds uncertainty and undermines learning. However, consistency need not mean rigidity. Contextual considerations and a child's intent can merit a calibrated response. The goal remains to cultivate virtue over punishment.

Reprimands are also teaching opportunities. Calmly explaining how an action fell short of expectations and its effects allows for reflection. Solutions can then be explored to make amends and apply the lesson elsewhere. Following through with natural consequences like the loss of privileges reinforces accountability. With consistency, boundaries become clear without requiring constant policing. Internalization takes root as respect, care, and responsibility towards self and others.

Transparently communicating expectations and behaviors lays the groundwork for comprehension and consistency. However, effective guidance is a two-way dialog where children also have a voice. Asking for their perspectives and checking to understand prevents assumptions. This builds trust for ongoing respectful exchanges. With practice, children gain confidence to bring concerns and appreciate multiple viewpoints.

Maintaining an open door invites discussing even difficult topics constructively. Young ones learn appropriate conduct through living examples as much as rules. Witnessing respectful conflict resolution in discussions models constructive problem-solving. Opportunities are created to practice these skills safely with guidance. In time, children internalize viewing others' humanity beyond external actions. This nurtures conduct upholding dignity in diverse real-world contexts ahead.

For children to embrace responsibility, appreciating the natural consequences of actions lays the foundation. Explanations linking behaviors to outcomes instill how to anticipate effects and take ownership. For instance, not completing chores on time could result in losing free time. Such teachings avoid harsh punitive approaches, instead illuminating cause and effect alignment. Children realize accountability strengthens trust while shirking it erodes relationships.

Opportunities to experience minor, safe failures encourage learning through trial. Calmly exploring what could have been done differently fosters responsibility versus resentment. Major lapses require corrective patience, but also restoring dignity. The aim remains to cultivate wiser choices versus instilling fear. With experience, children grasp outcomes stem intrinsically from within rather than externally imposed suffering. This nurtures independence balanced with care for communal well-being.

To feel invested in responsibility, having worthwhile roles tailored to capability aids engagement. Domestic tasks, schoolwork, or volunteer responsibilities lend purpose. However, roles respond to what inspires rather than forces involvement. Excessive or developmentally inappropriate demands risk resentment versus empowerment. Appropriate roles evolve as skills and maturity increase.

Likewise, lessening assistance gradually transfers ownership. Too quick a transition risks setbacks, while unlimited support delays growth. Calibrating challenge to competence nourishes responsibility and confidence. Roles also respect interests to align motivation over duty. Periodic reviews note accomplishments and readiness for expanded participation. This cultivates independent initiative balanced with reliance in times of need.

To internalize accountability, children require understanding the implications of inaction or neglect regarding duties, health, and safety. Potential risks of different scenarios provide perspective. However, a balance exists between prudent reflection and instilling chronic anxiety. The aim remains to cultivate wise choices through experience versus fear-based compliance.

For lapses minor in scale, natural consequences like re-doing tasks themselves encourage learning accountability. For more serious issues, calm discussions on mitigating risks in the future empower change. Blame serves no purpose versus insight gained. With guidance, children discern relying on others limits independent resilience shouldered through responsible choices. This nurtures both self-care and care for the community.

From safe failures emerges resilience enabling children to navigate complexities ahead. Sheltering denies learning how to pick oneself up and try anew. However, not all mistakes warrant the same learning. Distinguishing errors of judgment from negligence or recklessness prevents excusing preventable harm.

Minor stumbles serve as opportunities to problem-solve potential improvements calmly. For larger failures, validate feelings yet note growth demands reflection on responsibility. Rebuilding trust involves making amends independently. Children grasp independence necessitates resilience and accountability alongside support systems. This cultivates confidence in navigating life's uncertainties with empathy, care, and fortitude.

Gradually transferring ownership of responsibilities prepares children for self-reliance. However, independence progresses alongside nurturing trust and communal ties. Complete detachment risks losing balance. Interdependence honors relying on the supports available, without negating resilience strengthened through accountability.

As assumptions transfer, celebrations acknowledge the progress made. Challenges stem naturally from complexity versus arbitrary demands. With experience handling responsibilities matching capabilities, confidence blossoms in abilities to direct oneself and positively impact others. Independence thus cultivates through relationships marked by trust, care, and respect on the personal journey ahead navigating life's realities.

While boundaries, behavior guidance, and accountability cultivation each emphasize discrete developmental requisites, their synergistic significance emerges upon holistic contemplation.

Boundaries establish parameters wherein children may navigate relational intricacies and internalize responsibility for actions and their correlates, learning self-management indispensable for mature relationships and life participation. By outlining physical, emotional, and social boundaries age-appropriately clarified and consistently maintained, children internalize safety understanding and esteem-building self-awareness. Establishing boundaries early precludes later disorder and orientates development toward psyche-stabilizing independence.

Complementary to boundaries, behavior guidance conveys values and expectations which, when clarified and reinforced collaboratively between trusted figures and developing minds, nurture virtue internalization removing reliance on external motivation. Clarifying acceptability permits children to comprehend goodness as self-driven rather than imposed, empowering autonomy and conscience formation. Consistency therein inspires confidence that goodness reliably guides one's steps, relieving uncertainty that corrals potential.

Reinforcing accountable independence through natural consequence experience completes the triad, facilitating empathy cultivation and responsibility embodiment. By understanding actions shape experiences encouraging reflection rather than reaction, children cultivate perspective and diligence benefits. Allowing controlled mistakes within safe parameters permits challenge-emerged resilience strengthening, better preparing for complexity's inevitable encounters. Focus shifts from commands and consequences toward autonomous navigation informed by internalized lessons.

Collectively, these developmental architectures construct a fortress of mental fortitude. Rather than reacting to tribulations, children strengthened therein proactively confront complexities and forge purpose from perceptions. External discipline transmutes to self-mastery as internal guidance supersedes dependence. Resilience, forged through experience within conscientious boundaries of safety and virtue, fortifies against difficulty's corrosion. Confidence blossoms as competence grows from empowered autonomy rather than external reward-seeking. Relationships flourish on mutual understanding rather than control.

While boundaries, behavior clarity, and accountability each emphasize a developmental virtue, their unity constructs a cohesive and self-sustaining edifice of strength. Neither commanding obedience nor permissiveness, this balanced approach nurtures autonomy and conscience in companionship. Children learn relationships sustain rather than constrain potentials as self-discipline supplants willfulness. Hardship enhances wisdom rather than wounding spirit. Life emerges as an adventure rather than an obstacle course as internal drives eclipse external validation-seeking.

This integrated developmental orchestration cultivates dignified sophistication enabling engaged life participation. Rather than surviving tribulations, lives may be crafted and challenges met with perspective, diligence, and community. Suffering loses sting as resilience buffers its cutting wind. Purpose emerges intuitively from conscience informed by experience within parameters of cultivated virtue. Lives unfold as creative journeys emerging from strength of character rather than wayward circumstances. Society flourishes as individuals contribute fruits ripened on the balanced developmental vine wherein understanding, courage and compassion intertwine.

While boundaries, behavior guidance, and accountability directly cultivate certain strengths, their unity constructs a self-sustaining framework elevating perspectives, relationships, and life potentials. Lives shaped herein emerge empowered to craft purpose and meaning from complex encounters, experiencing adventure wherein challenges enhance rather than deter life's unfolding blossom. May our efforts uplift not only children but through their influence better worlds wherein dignity, courage, and community flourish for all.

Problem-Solving Skills

Life presents humans with obstacles both large and small daily. Successfully overcoming challenges requires more than just reacting - it demands careful consideration and thoughtful action. Developing strong problem-solving abilities equips individuals with a powerful toolkit to navigate adversity and achieve goals. Problem-solving skills have value across all domains of life, from academics and careers to relationships and well-being. No matter the specific problem at hand, a measured, strategic approach can help one arrive at effective solutions.

Education frequently relies on problem-solving as a core learning process. From tackling math word problems to analyzing literary themes, students must employ deduction, logical reasoning, and creative thinking to move past roadblocks. Strong problem-solving skills facilitate deeper engagement with course material and lead to superior understanding. Identifying the crux of an academic issue allows learners to break it down into manageable parts and methodically explore potential answers. Developing multiple hypotheses, testing theories, and reflecting on outcomes cultivate intellectually agile students well-positioned for ongoing challenges. Problem-solving also transfers readily to other domains - these cross-context skills prove invaluable for independent study, open-inquiry projects, and tackling complex assignments beyond the classroom. Maintaining an analytical, systematic approach to difficulties supports academic achievement now and serves lifelong learning.

The contemporary workforce demands flexible, autonomous thinkers who can effectively troubleshoot, prioritize tasks, and generate innovative solutions. Problem-solving provides a competitive edge for any career path. It allows professionals to adeptly manage responsibilities, embrace multifaceted duties, and navigate obstacles that arise unexpectedly. Strong problem-solvers showcase versatile intelligence appreciated by employers; they analyze multifaceted issues from a big-picture vantage point while attentive to important subtleties. Tackling difficulties with composure, efficiency, and resourcefulness fosters a productive work climate. Problem-solving furthermore grounds continuous self-improvement - soliciting feedback from setbacks breeds ongoing refinement. Staying stalwart yet adaptive futureproofs careers navigating unpredictable technological and socioeconomic terrain. Cultivating this skill set enhances job performance, career mobility, and opportunities for leadership over the long run.

Interpersonal relationships constantly present dilemmas both large and small. Problem-solving smooths social interactions by facilitating compromise during conflicts and debates. It hones listening skills, empathy for others' perspectives, and compromise - pillars of healthy bonds. Approaching relationship difficulties thoughtfully through open communication and patience prevents misunderstandings from festering. Problem-solving further fosters social-emotional intelligence, building self-awareness and regulating strong reactions that could damage ties. It nurtures compassion by encouraging examination of others' motives and life experiences contributing to issues. This capability to objectively yet caringly work through interpersonal challenges proves invaluable for family dynamics, partnerships, and social circles of all kinds. While disagreements may arise, problem-solving ensures the well-being of connections above all else.

Life presents unavoidable hardships that demand perseverance despite setbacks. Problem-solving cultivates resilience by encouraging confronting difficulties with empathy, responsibility, and growth-focused perseverance. It fosters realism about inevitable obstacles while retaining optimism that issues can be managed if not always perfectly solved. Approaching problems systematically discourages all-or-nothing thinking and compulsive avoidance behaviors that undermine well-being. Breaking down large stresses into smaller, actionable components relieves overwhelm and motivates continued progress. Looking back and appreciating growth from past hurdles bolsters confidence to weather ongoing struggles. Handling difficulties with patience, diligence, and flexibility prevents catastrophizing failures and reacting harshly to minor slip-ups. Ultimately, problem-solving anchors resilience by validating the inherent human capacity for overcoming hardship through perseverance, insight, and community support.

Fortunately, problem-solving skills can be intentionally developed at any life stage through dedication and practice. Some effective strategies include:

Maintaining a journal to document obstacles encountered and contemplated solutions over time. Reflect on what worked well and identify areas for improvement.

Deliberately seeking out open-ended, complex challenges requiring multifaceted thinking rather than single-step fixes. Consciously break down large issues into smaller, more manageable pieces for systematic exploration. Actively listen to understand all facets of problems presented, brainstorming diverse perspectives without judgment. Question initial assumptions to avoid premature conclusions.

When stuck, take breaks to relieve mental fatigue before reapproaching with a fresh lens. Clear mindsets allow novel ideas to emerge.

Practice "thinking out loud" to trace logical trains of thought. Discover gaps or logical leaps needing rationale. Modify approaches based on insightful feedback.

Study models of elite problem-solvers across disciplines, noting versatile techniques and perseverance despite setbacks. Emulate inquiry, diligence, and resilience.

Remind oneself that problems are solvable through patience and community. Seek insight from others to stimulate creativity when energy wavers.

Celebrate both successes and instructive failures with equal gratitude for the learning. Revel in continued self-refinement over time.

Problem-solving skills empower individuals to maintain poise and productivity despite obstacles through logical, comprehensive processes. These transferable abilities prove invaluable across academics, careers, relationships, and personal well-being. With dedicated practice over time, problem-solving grows into a versatile core strength supporting consistent achievement and fulfilling experiences. Ultimately, it anchors resilience by validating inherent human capacities for facing hardship with patience, empathy, creativity, and community support. Life's complexities simply deserve thoughtful, multifaceted solutions.

Disagreements often emerge from sharing limited resources like toys. Children respectively want their way and haven't fully developed patience or compromise. Additional friction points involve misunderstandings, hurt feelings, accusations of unfairness, and conflicting needs for attention or control in activities. Playground disputes additionally arise from miscommunications and struggles over physical boundaries or imagined slights. Preteen conflicts may relate to inclusion dramas, romantic tensions, or attempts to assert independence by testing previous alliances. Adults must embrace each developmental stage's complex social dynamics to coach nuanced resolutions.

Learning to thoughtfully work through disagreements benefits kids tremendously. It builds communication skills, perspective-taking, and complex problem-solving applicable in myriad contexts. Children better understand actions impacting others and how to repair fractured relationships. Resolving issues respectfully and cooperatively models fulfilling interactions children will seek throughout life. It fosters self-awareness to identify and regulate intense emotions constructively. Navigating conflicts supports strong peer relationships central to well-being, bolstering self-esteem, and preventing depression or anxiety relating to social stressors. Children anchored in mutual understanding resolution techniques navigate teenage and adult dilemmas with greater poise and care for all perspectives. Addressing disputes proactively and non-judgmentally maximizes social-emotional gains.

Staying calm and solutions-focused sets the tone for productive discussion. Listen actively and reflect on feelings to validate all perspectives before suggesting resolutions. Questions can uncover motivations respectfully, and paraphrasing prevents assumptions. Drawing connections between actions and feelings prevents blaming, focusing on impacts and solutions.

Brainstorm possible solutions together, considering the interests driving each friend's position. For younger children, model techniques through role plays demonstrate understanding, patience, and care for relationships over desires in the moment. Compromise allows various viewpoints, finding flexibility children can feel positively about.

Celebrating cooperation affirms children's hard work in navigating difficulties respectfully. Reminders that strong friendships sometimes include misunderstandings, and kindness overcomes all, help sustain resolutions. Monitoring agreements and supporting accountability reinforces skills, and reminding to come to adults if conflicts resume prevents issues from festering.

For toddlers and preschoolers, address conflicts gently amid play to maintain engagement. Name feelings simply, avoid complex questioning, and suggest resolutions with tangible actions. Praise respect, compromise, and use "kind words."

In elementary grades, children gain perspective-taking skills. Ask what happened from each friend's viewpoint without interruption. Paraphrase feelings and brainstorm multiple solutions agreeable to both.

For preteens, respect the privacy of resolution where reasonable, and provide guidance when requested. Remind disagreements happen even among close friends, and cooperation strengthens bonds long-term despite momentary tensions.

Across developmental stages, withholding judgment, focusing on respect, and valuing relationships over short-term wins cultivate skills serving children wherever life's complex journey may lead. While disagreements arise, addressing them consistently yet caringly establishes a foundation for fulfillment.

Beyond individual conflicts, additional techniques support social-emotional development:

Foster communicating feelings through journaling, interactive apps or role plays to build self-awareness and expression.

Engage in regular family meetings to discuss challenges, share gratitude, and bring conflicts constructively.

Suggest compromise activities all children enjoy, emphasizing cooperation and consideration for others' interests.

Model and discuss acts of kindness, cheering accomplishments, and saying "I'm sorry" when mistakes are made.

Affirm identity and independence while reminding of caregivers' constant support through all of life's ups and downs.

Limit technology interfering with social interactions, instead encouraging creative play developing empathy and perspective-taking.

With guidance and leading by example, children internalize resolving conflicts respectfully. Prioritizing relationships over desires in any given moment and finding flexibility cultivates fulfilling social skills. While problems inevitably emerge alongside lessons, a foundation of care, respect, and mutual understanding established early on supports children's capacity for resilient, compassionate navigation of life's complex dynamics. Prioritizing these interpersonal virtues above individual aims maximizes social and emotional growth for years to come.

Compromise validates all viewpoints rather than dismissing some as wrong. It finds common ground allowing give-and-take to satisfy core concerns driving initial positions. Relationships require cooperation navigating life's complexities respectfully. Compromise respects this inherently, relinquishing full desires for relationships' greater benefit. It models seeing beyond one's wants to others' humanity as the resolution's guiding light. Creative solutions exist strengthening all sides' positions rather than validating one outright at others' expense. Compromise nurtures flexibility crucial to navigation's unexpected terrain shifts, building trust to weather inevitable future disagreements. While initial desire may differ from the negotiated outcome, goodwill maintained salvages dignity on all sides.

Empathy provides the scaffolding for workable compromise by humanizing differing viewpoints. It prompts suspending assumptions to hear all perspectives fully with a non-judgmental presence. Only by deeply comprehending others' motivations and experiences can cooperative resolutions honor humanity in all involved. Paraphrasing reflects this understanding, validating emotional truths at conflicts' roots and preventing invalidation from fueling resentment. Addressing not just behaviors but their impacts nurtures care, accountability, and repair over defensiveness. Comprehending complexity discourages reductionism, leaving room for grace and second chances as relationships living, evolving entities. Ultimately, empathy transforms adversaries into allies working as a team toward harmonious solutions.

Compassion and understanding prove especially vital among close relationships weathering life together. Flexibility maintains their comfort through inevitable tensions instead of risking fracture. Partners share emotional truths lovingly to strengthen intimacy rather than "winning" debates. Families embrace a spectrum of perspectives to nurture unity against diversity. Friends grant leeway acknowledging nobody's perfect while prioritizing bonds' longevity. The resolution affirms relationships' importance above momentary desires, embracing vulnerability to repair misunderstandings before they take root. The compromise here cultivates security to weather hardships collaboratively, empathy transforming issues into opportunities bolstering care, respect, and trust sustaining connections through all upcoming challenges.

Resolutions begin by explicitly stating the desire for mutually agreeable solutions respecting all involved, ensuring composure prevails. Listen intently to comprehend core interests and perspectives completely before advocating one's viewpoint. Affirm humanity and relationship importance above individual positions. Discuss alternatives meeting as many interests as possible; brainstorming creatively without judgment unlocks novel solutions. Negotiate adjustments collaboratively and finalize agreements cementing goodwill. Revisit understandings occasionally to prevent resentments. Though challenges remain, maintaining positivity and forgiveness anchors resolutions maintaining dignity and care on all sides.

Overcoming Resistance to Compromise Nature can resist compromise from ingrained attitudes like perfectionism, rigidity, or scarcity mindsets preventing flexibility. However, understanding perspective shifts can motivate change. Recognizing life's uncertainties, interdependence, and diversity of viewpoints validates our inherent fallibility. No solution perfectly satisfies all sides, yet relationships remain worth flexible cooperation. Reframing compromise as creative problem-solving dignifies all voices. Additionally, reflecting on relationships nurturing our well-being inspires reciprocity and willingness to meet others partway. Ultimately, openness and willingness to grow together compassionately transform even historically aversive situations.

As life presents complexities, flexibility and care for humanity in all its diversity prove resolution's surest guides. Compromise and understanding maintain dignity while cultivating cooperation through empathy, nuanced listening, and creative give-and-take. Small acts of goodwill weather daily interactions, while larger displays reinforce commitments through difficulties. Ultimately, prioritizing relationships anchors personal and collective well-being by recognizing our inherent interconnectedness. Resolutions become not ends but means nurturing care, trust, and fulfillment together into the future.

Problem-solving skills are engendered by methodical consideration of obstacles, extraction of layered significances, and discovery of resourceful options, building resilience as children learn defiance of circumstance through their ingenious efforts. Conflict resolution proceeds apace, as interpersonal difficulties arise providing opportunities to practice empathetic understanding and mutually agreeable solutions - invaluable lessons translatable to life's tapestry of relationships. Compromise embodied here, as opposing perspectives reconciled for shared benefit, lays the foundations for principled cooperation certain to complexity's inevitable encounters.

Together, these developmental bastions fortify young minds against tumult through the cultivation of perspective, courage, and community-orienting lives outward from turmoil rather than defined by it. Children emerge better equipped to craft purpose and meaning even amid discrepant experiences, as internal strengths outshine transient discords sure to arise. Problem-solving cultivated individual empowerment as resourcefulness supplanted vulnerability; conflict navigation nurtured social refinement through understanding rather than dominance; compromise constructed frameworks for principled accord where diverse views enrich collective welfare.

A cohesive developmental tapestry emerges, distinctly alternative to perspectives of coping versus thriving. Here, challenges exist not to be survived but overcome, with wisdom and relationships reinforced in the process. Resilience buffers life's irregularities rather than succumbing to external dictates. Purpose intuitively arises from virtue internalized through such fortifying experiences, navigated with vigor, nuance, and community.

We reflect on the potential societal fruits borne of such an integrated developmental approach. While individual strengths like resolve, tact, and cooperation emerge initially, gifts thus cultivated portend humankind uplifted - sharing adventures wherein diversity enriches common pursuits of dignity. May our shared work nourish not only youth but worlds awakened to life's grandeur through courage, understanding, and accord and liberated thereby to flourish. Our investments today herald tomorrow's blossoms.

Independence and Self-Reliance

Encouraging independence in children from an early age plays a significant role in their overall development and prepares them for adulthood. Allowing children to try accomplishing tasks and solving problems on their own instills vital life skills and traits that serve them well into the future. While providing guidance and support as needed, parents and caregivers need to give age-appropriate freedom and responsibilities to children to foster self-reliance. Doing so helps nurture independence, resilience, responsibility, decision-making skills, and other attributes critical for success.

One of the primary advantages of fostering independence is that it helps children develop important lifelong skills. When allowed to take on responsibilities and small tasks matched to their abilities, kids learn practical competencies like completing chores, following schedules, managing money, preparing basic meals, and more. They also gain problem-solving acumen as they figure out creative solutions when facing obstacles independently. Additionally, fostering independence enables children to hone decision-making skills through practicing making choices on daily matters like clothing, after-school activities, and homework routines. It also strengthens critical thinking as kids learn to weigh different options and consider the causes and consequences of decisions. All these skills set the foundation for navigating more complex responsibilities and challenges as children grow.

Another significant benefit of granting children age-appropriate independence is that it boosts their self-confidence and self-esteem over time. When given opportunities to accomplish tasks and make decisions independently, kids derive a sense of pride, competence, and achievement from their efforts. Mastering new skills and responsibilities alone fuels confidence in one's abilities. Additionally, allowing mistakes sans judgment and providing praise and acknowledgment for efforts nurtures confidence even when challenges occur. Children gradually learn they possess the agency to tackle issues and assert their autonomy. This lays the groundwork for possessing robust self-belief and the courage to explore interests freely as they mature. High self-esteem, in turn, protects independence and enables kids to advocate for themselves positively.

Perhaps one of the most important life qualities cultivated through independence is resilience - the ability to withstand and rebound from difficulties, setbacks, and life's uncertainties. When children are given freedom matched to their developmental levels to make errors and find solutions alone, they gain insight into persevering through obstacles. Experiencing minor failures helps kids develop a growth mindset to learn from experiences rather than face defeat. It also fosters adaptability as children learn various methods to overcome challenges through self-directed efforts. Over time, kids become more equipped to withstand larger setbacks and transitions with tenacity, optimism, and flexibility. This helps lay the foundation for shrugging off life's inevitable curveballs with poise, faith in one's abilities, and the tools to spring back quickly.

In addition to skill-building and emotional learning, cultivating independence aids in instilling a strong sense of responsibility in children from an early age. When granted self-reliance through chores, homework habits, and daily tasks, kids realize their actions and choices impact not just themselves but also others around them. With experience, they understand they are accountable for following through consistently and making wise decisions with little oversight. This helps children develop critical perspectives like responsibility for one's health, safety, decisions, family duties, and more. It also supports integrity as kids practice dependability. Nurturing responsibility better equips children to manage their obligations independently and make considerate choices with society's best interests in mind as they mature.

Another advantage of fostering independence is that it encourages creativity, curiosity, and innovative thinking in children. When given the freedom to explore passions and handle challenges without undue structure or expectations, kids are more inclined to take risks, think outside the box, and devise novel solutions on their own terms. Independence nurtures a sense of inner drive and enthusiasm to investigate new possibilities. It also instills confidence to experiment, learn from failures, and bravely pursue aspirations regardless of potential disapproval from others. Over time, this flexes critical and conceptual thinking muscles to tackle issues innovatively. It inspires kids to freely contribute their quirky ideas, follow unconventional strategies, and think ambitiously about the future with fewer self-imposed limitations.

One of the primary advantages of allowing choices and consequences is the hands-on learning it facilitates. As children test decision-making muscles, they gain insight directly from the results. This cements lessons more profoundly than detached advice. For example, a child may choose an ambitious school project and feel tired from the workload, so learning time management is important. Or they may pick an unhealthy breakfast and feel sluggish, gaining a nutrition perspective. While protecting from serious harm, permitting experiential education equips kids to learn from small wins and errors alike. It cultivates a growth mindset valuing lessons over outcomes and inspires tenacity to grow from missteps.

Another benefit is fostering personal accountability as children discern choice impacts. Experiencing positive and negative consequences anchors the connection between actions and results. For instance, a child selecting an earlier bedtime may feel well-rested and focus on understanding that sequence. In contrast, one who chooses electronics past bedtime may feel consequences like grumpiness, reinforcing responsibility for self-care. Growing up with natural outcomes promotes conscientious decision-making respectful of how choices affect both oneself and others. It empowers kids to make wise choices aligned with their well-being and responsibilities rather than shirking accountability.

Allowing choices and consequences also strengthens children's problem-solving muscles. Facing decisions with autonomous yet supportive navigation of results flexes adaptive thinking. For example, a child may choose an excessively challenging project, feel overwhelmed, and learn to pace work better next time. Or one who forgets lunch money may face hunger pangs and brainstorm reliable backup plans. With experience navigating dilemmas independently, kids become more resourceful, flexible problem-solvers adept at learning from missteps. They enhance abilities to assess situations, devise strategies, implement solutions, and adjust approaches for varied conditions.

Furthermore, granting choices provides opportunities to develop perspective-taking skills. As children observe how choices affect themselves, they simultaneously gain insight into how decisions impact others. For instance, a child who chooses not to complete chores may better understand how that decision burdens family members tasked with extra work. One who opts out of teamwork may recognize the feelings of teammates who must adjust plans. Experiencing consequences firsthand cultivates humility, consideration, and care for others challenged by one's actions. It nurtures empathy for differing perspectives and situations outside of oneself.

A key benefit of allowing choices is imparting decision-making acumen itself. Through guided practice considering options, children become more adept at contemplating pros and cons, potential outcomes, and responsibilities inherent in various alternatives. They gain familiarity with thinking through complexities and assessing the short and long-term implications of decisions. With experience and feedback, kids enhance their abilities to make careful, well-reasoned choices aligned with priorities like ethics, commitments, and personal growth. They learn cognitive skills useful for navigating everyday decisions and also weightier life intersections.

While choices provide rich learning, guidance supports child development. Some suggestions:

Provide age-appropriate options respecting safety, values, and abilities. Avoid overwhelming complexity.

Discuss thoughts and feelings respectfully around possible choices to cultivate discernment.

For younger children, involve them in some decision aspects like choosing clothes for the identified context.

Clarify natural connections between choices and ensuing realities or assistance available.

Respect choice outcome whether initially preferred or not; revisit factors to glean learning, not assign blame.

Periodically check in on choice experiences, noting lessons and discussing how insights may influence future decisions.

Respect developing independence while maintaining oversight to ensure well-being and habits supporting responsibilities.

One way to foster self-motivation is to emphasize intrinsic rather than extrinsic motivation. Intrinsic factors like interests, goals, challenges, or learning itself fuel internal drive, as opposed to external rewards like praise or privileges. Research shows intrinsic motivation correlates more closely with academic performance and long-term achievement. While occasional praise can encourage effort, relying too heavily on extrinsic factors can diminish self-determination over time. Focusing instead on cultivating natural curiosity, mastery, and perseverance cultivates lifelong self-motivation.

Teaching goal-setting provides structure supporting self-motivation and discipline. Goals should be specific, measurable, attainable, relevant, and time-bound (SMART) to facilitate focus. Younger children may set goals like reading for 10 minutes daily or practicing an instrument, while older kids focus on projects, grades, or responsibilities. Celebrating small wins and adjusting as needed keeps goals challenging yet achievable. Breaking larger goals into steps also supports follow-through. Periodic check-ins on progress, not just results, further nurture intrinsic drive through effort acknowledgment.

Fostering a growth rather than a fixed mindset cultivates resilience crucial for self-motivation. With a growth mindset, abilities grow through dedication rather than being predetermined. Mistakes are viewed as learning opportunities rather than failures, inspiring perseverance through setbacks. Praise emphasizes effort, strategies, and improvement rather than intellect to encourage experimenting beyond comfort zones. Modeling and discussing overcoming personal setbacks through strategies like help-seeking, revising plans, or focusing on progress, not perfection can cultivate this empowering perspective.

Consistently applying techniques supports developing discipline. Establishing routines for organizing time and responsibilities with checklists, calendars or reminders promotes follow-through habits. Recognizing and avoiding distractions through designated study areas and technology downtimes also bolsters focus. Sleeping, nutrition, exercise, and stress management promote well-being facilitating discipline. Limiting choices or removing non-essentials when overwhelmed prevents options paralysis. Accountability through discussion and goal-tracking helps identify motivators and obstacles to continuously strengthen discipline.

Self-awareness underpins self-motivation and discipline. Children can reflect on strengths, areas for growth, and stressors through journals. Recognizing personal responsibility for results rather than blaming external factors fosters internal locus of control. For example, prioritizing challenging assignment sections or employing new focus methods acknowledges agency over outcomes. Responsibility also involves self-care, honesty, and upholding commitments. Striving to meet expectations through perseverance despite distress acknowledges room for growth and willingness to push limits.

While independence develops by navigating challenges, interdependence remains important. Expressing struggle productively to parents or role models allows brainstorming solutions to strengthen resolve. Mentors can attest to overcoming disappointments and motivating ongoing efforts. Peers can form study groups enhancing accountability and inspiration through collaboration. Role models like diligent historical figures evoke vicarious motivation through hardship and triumph. Communities provide resources like tutoring, counseling, or activities sustaining passion. Ultimately, self-motivation and discipline result from nurturing strengths through adversity within supportive networks.

Fostering independence establishes appreciation that potential emergence arises through dedicated action rather than transient circumstances. Problem-solving, initiated through opportunities to navigate undertakings freely, cultivates resourcefulness enabling challenges overcome. Self-confidence buds as competence grows from experience.

Allowing choice experience and subsequent consequence orientation reinforces the above, as accountability emerges from within through direct discovery that decisions bear ramifications requiring sagacious consideration. Perspective broadens in empathy's cultivation along autonomy's path. Wisdom blossoms where willfulness once reigned.

Self-motivation and discipline's encouragement comprise the apex of this developmental edifice, wherein lives may be crafted purposefully through dedication to the purposeful actualization of inherently worthwhile potentials. Intrinsic drives supplant reliance on fleeting reward dynamics, empowering persistently vigorous pursuit amid inevitable difficulties. Growth orientation nourishes optimism that greater heights emerge through efforts, however modest initially.

Collectively, these developmental bastions shape lives inclined intrinsically toward betterment and achievement through virtue of character rather than reaction to circumstance. Resilience shields against complexity's natural irregularities as confidence arises from within, nourishing adventurous life participation from a place of fortified dignity. Creativity flourishes where rules once constrained, empowering innovation's fruits. Purpose intuitively emerges for dynamic contribution wherein diversity enriches collaborative equity.

Relationships prosper on mutual empowerment rather than domination, as understanding exceeds enforcement. Societal well-being arises organically from individuals thus oriented. Though challenges remain, perspectives shift from constraints to be endured, to adventures wherein triumph springs from cultivated strengths driving lives of meaning, vigor, and community. Our shared work today heralds this promise, and generations shaped by wisdom to follow.

Gratitude and Positivity

Gratitude is a thankful appreciation for what one has. It involves actively acknowledging the people, health, opportunities, and experiences in our lives that contribute value and meaning, rather than passively and perhaps negatively focusing on what is lacking. Feeling grateful doesn't mean ignoring life's challenges but having the perspective that many aspects of our existence are blessings despite imperfections. Research defines two aspects of gratitude - feelings of appreciation and being able to acknowledge sources of benefits. While appreciation involves an affective sense of thankfulness, acknowledgment taps cognitive understanding of external contributions. Both components interact in a reciprocal relationship cultivated through regular practice.

Cultivating gratitude yields a multitude of well-documented positive psychological impacts with implications for preventing and treating mental illnesses. Studies have linked gratitude to greater happiness and life satisfaction through reduced materialism and healthier social comparisons. It is associated with less depression and stress due to a more optimistic outlook and perspective on challenges as temporary rather than permanent. Gratitude may diminish anxiety by enhancing gratitude's link to savoring life's beauty and meaning rather than worrying excessively. Expressing appreciation to others also strengthens relationship well-being and social support imperative for mental hygiene. Feeling grateful impacts cognitive processes like sleep, decision-making, and rumination in more productive ways bolstering overall resilience too.

Research specifically correlates gratitude deficiencies to increased depression, anxiety, post-traumatic stress disorder (PTSD), and substance abuse. For example, counting blessings is associated with decreased depression symptoms more than focusing on justice, self-improvement, or daily activities.

One study found individuals praising others reduced cortisol stress levels similar to anti-anxiety medications without side effects. Sharing gratitude also seems beneficial for trauma recovery, likely due to social bonding and reduced feelings of threat. Conversely, gratitude interventions show promise for relapse prevention among recovering addicts through fostering non-materialistic pleasures and closer community ties countering substance dependence. Overall, cultivating thankfulness appears a protective mental health attribute.

Given research support, intentionally nurturing gratitude using structured practices can greatly benefit emotional and physical well-being. Here are some effective suggestions:

Keep a daily gratitude journal, writing down 3-6 things appreciated each evening for longevity.

Verbalize thankfulness through thank-you calls, cards, or in-person expressions for enhanced social bonding.

Practice gratitude meditations focusing on gratitude, its sources, and its impact for sustained positive focus.

Involve friends and family via gratitude discussions facilitating understanding and care between relationships.

Celebrate blessings through cultural traditions honoring what matters mentally, spiritually, or culturally.

Mindfully savor life's simple pleasures through a slowed focus on beauty, flavors, and sensations with present-moment awareness. Reframe setbacks and embrace non-perfectionism through growth rather than a fixed mindset nurturing resilience and well-being despite hardships.

Incorporating regular, mindful gratitude elevates happiness, compassion, and general optimism through a switch to strengths-based, present-moment awareness nourishing mental wellness.

While life inevitably presents difficulties, maintaining a positive mental attitude can significantly impact well-being, success, and quality of relationships. Optimism involves expecting favorable outcomes and believing challenges can be overcome through perseverance and available resources. Research shows a positive mindset benefits mental, emotional, and even physical health through reduced stress, stronger immune functioning, and healthier behaviors. Optimists also tend to have richer social ties and successfully reach life goals through grit and creative problem-solving.

A positive mindset is an inclination towards an upbeat perspective despite setbacks or uncertainties. Rather than negativity bias gravitating toward threats, an optimist embraces opportunities and sees the glass as half full. They focus on progress and solutions by addressing controllable factors, letting uncontrollable elements roll off more easily through resilience. Optimism is built on expecting desirable results from efforts and trusting the capability to handle difficulties through support systems if needed. It involves flexibility remaining open to outcomes while retaining drive and navigating obstacles resourcefully. A positive mindset takes time to train but greatly impacts well-being, relationships, and achievements through proactive problem-solving.

Maintaining optimism yields profound psychological advantages and physical health correlations according to scientific research:

Optimists have increased happiness, life satisfaction, and subjective well-being due to positive perceptions rather than denial of difficulties.

Optimism promotes proactive coping through tenacious goal-pursuit rather than avoidance of obstacles boosting performance and accomplishments.

Resilient thinking supports healthy stress response, diminishing cortisol release and enhancing immunity through impactful lifestyle behaviors like nutrition, activity, and rest.

A positive outlook fosters richer relationships via empathy, support-seeking, and care for others rather than isolation, building social resources vital for well-being.

Optimism facilitates perseverance enabling setback transcendence and intrinsic motivation facing challenges independently yet cooperatively too.

An optimistic cognitive style may correlate to healthier biomarker profiles implicating retarded cellular aging and lower disease risk over the lifespan.

Several strategies can foster an optimistic mindset with practice and persistence:

Notice and reframe unhelpful negative self-talk by acknowledging the good without denying difficulties and flexibility for changes.

Practice gratitude daily through journaling blessings in life to activate prefrontal positivity and resilience neural pathways countering pessimism.

Set achievable, specific goals and break them into bite-sized tasks focusing on progress rather than perfection through diligence.

Nurture optimism in others via modeling upbeat problem-solving, acts of kindness, and validating people's best intentions and humanity.

Limit exposure to toxic news skewing toward threats replacing it with uplifting content fueling inspiration.

Self-care properly through sleep, nutrition, relaxation, and modest pleasures keeps the mind engaged in living fully.

Remember past successes navigating setbacks through considered strategies, resilience, and community rather than weakness alone.

Cultivate intrinsic motivations and interests fueling internal purpose countering dependency on unstable external factors.

Challenge absolutist thinking open to growth from both wins and losses with humility and flexibility rather than rigidity and conclusions.

Be mindful of present moments detracting from regrets/worries and focus on progressive improvements daily through perseverance.

Nurture supportive relationships uplifting each other cooperatively rather than enabling defeatism detrimental to wellness.

Express optimism for others through acts of service releasing oxytocin facilitating positive emotional contagion strengthening social bonds.

Optimism is not denial but realistic hope balancing challenge and opportunity through diligent, resourceful problem-solving enriching quality of life at both individual and collective levels as an adaptive mindset disposition. Regularly practicing optimistic strategies leverages well-being and success potential across diverse life domains.

Maintaining a positive outlook also proves vital for self-actualization and enrichment. Optimism fuels curiosity exploring interests boosting fulfillment. It inspires embracing weaknesses as learning and refining strengths through patience. Optimistic self-reflection involves humbly processing both virtues and blind spots non-judgmentally desiring improvement. Appreciating progress along an integrity-aligned purpose nourishes well-being far beyond fleeting pleasures. Optimism generates tenacity in navigating identity stages cooperatively while retaining freedom facilitating autonomous adulthood. It motivates passing wisdom gained from hardships to uplift others indicating maturity. Most importantly, optimism anchors adaptability navigating uncertainties with poise, faith in humanity, and commitment to becoming the best versions of selves amid life's shifting conditions.

Optimism proves more than a subjective perspective but a self-fulfilling, learnable proposition correlated to enhanced health, achievement, relationships, and personal evolution. While regularly facing difficulties, a positive mindset cultivates resilience and focuses on opportunities through diligence rather than denial or passivity. Optimism transforms setbacks into growth and fuels perseverance independently yet interdependently alongside the community. It anchors present well-being and longevity through rich involvement and purpose navigating life's complex terrain resourcefully, cooperatively, and with poise. With practice and perspective, optimism facilitates thriving amid both joys and inevitable hardships.

Gratitude cultivation, by orienting perspectives outward to life's fleeting beauties rather than inward to perceived deficiencies, nurtures perseverant optimism even amid difficulty. Studies corroborating well-being improvements illuminate gratitude's crucial role in maintaining mental soundness. Yet deeper insight arises - through appreciation of each gracious moment does purpose find affirmation, revitalizing determination's flame within.

Encouraging grateful appreciation in developing minds anchors this foundation, as youth learn perspective broadening with experience. Relationships and character strengthen in empathy thus nurtured. Resilience grows where vulnerability once thrived, empowering lives bolstered to weather complexity's inevitable encounters. Appreciation becomes a lens emphasizing opportunities within hardships, ennobling purpose's emergence.

A positive outlook completes the developmental triad, wherein the focus shifts from perceived inadequacies to potentials warranted by past gifts and future dreams. Problem-solving and physical health excel where reactivity was once hindered. Self-reflection cultivated through gratitude and optimism nourishes continuing growth and contribution - an existence indeed worth living.

Together, these developmental currents forge lives inclined dynamically toward actualization and adventure. Resolve outpaces resignation as character surmounts circumstance. Creativity flourishes where rules once constrained, empowering innovation from hardship's lessons. Purpose intuitively emerges for meaningful participation in a shared, brightening future.

Physical Health

Maintaining good physical and mental health is essential for overall well-being and happiness. While modern society has become increasingly more sedentary, research conclusively links regular physical activity to improved psychological outcomes like reduced stress, anxiety, and depression symptoms. Exercise positively impacts brain chemistry, boosts self-esteem, and facilitates stress-coping strategies.

Several biological mechanisms explain exercise's powerful impact on mood and brain function. Physical activity stimulates the release of endorphins, the brain's natural painkillers, and feel-good chemicals like dopamine and serotonin that improve mood. It also increases the production of endocannabinoids boosting euphoria, relaxation, and appetite through pathways simulating cannabis albeit naturally without side effects. Exercise further reduces stress hormones like cortisol diminishing the cumulative wear and tear they cause when chronically elevated. Studies observe resulting structural changes in the hippocampus, a pivotal brain region for mood regulation, learning, and memory entrenching exercise's mental protections over the lifespan.

Substantial research now confirms regular physical activity significantly diminishes depression's severity compared to inactive lifestyles. Studies find just 30 minutes daily of moderate activity reduces symptoms as effectively as antidepressants for mild to moderate depression without side effects. Exercise improves mood through natural highs as previously discussed but also provides a healthy outlet for alleviating stress or distracting from ruminating thoughts. Cardio workouts in nature also present restoration boosting resilience against future vulnerability. Regarding anxiety, exercise strengthens self-efficacy and coping strategies diminishing physiological arousal from worries across disorders.

While most physical activities provide gains, some show unique advantages:

Aerobic exercise like running, dancing, or swimming strengthens the cardiovascular system boosting mood-lifting endorphins, endocannabinoids, and neuroplasticity in reward centers over time.

Weight training builds confidence through visible muscle and strength improvements crucial for self-image while reducing stress and tension.

Yoga joins breathing, stretching, and mindfulness calming activities providing relaxation while rejuvenating mobility.

Team sports facilitate camaraderie improving social wellness and a sense of purpose according to research on associated risks for mental illnesses declining with involvement. Outdoor exercise exposes individuals to microbes boosting immune function while sunset hormones like melatonin may induce better quality sleep through light exposure balance.

To harness the psychological benefits of exercise, consistency matters most. Aim for at least 150 minutes weekly spread over days suiting schedules through:

Walking meetings, stretching breaks, or using stationary cycles at work to pair movement with daily tasks.

Planning family excursions like hiking, swimming, court games, or bike rides makes exercise a fun group bonding activity.

Joining evening classes, jogging with a friend, or using fitness apps for virtual support and variety.

Performing strength exercises at home requiring no special equipment such as bodyweight squats and pushups.

Practicing relaxation activities before bed like gentle yoga, foam rolling, or reading in a bath to induce better sleep quality through a shift to parasympathetic function.

In addition to direct impacts on mental health, regular activity confers advantageous side benefits through:

Cardiorespiratory improvements lowering risks for heart disease, diabetes, and some cancers as top disease killers diminish mental burdens from health concerns.

Muscle and bone strengthening reduce injury likelihood and related depression symptoms from functionality losses too.

Lifelong habits inspire purpose providing structure for reliable coping strategies during difficulties.

Weight regulation boosts body image and self-esteem gains central for psychological wellness alongside interdependent physical health variables optimized through activity.

Stress resilience forms through setting and achieving exercise-related goals facilitating successes transferrable to wider life domains too.

Getting children involved in sports and physical activities pays rich developmental dividends impacting both the body and mind. While sedentary habits now displace movement for many youths, studies show exercise enhances concentration, self-esteem, teamwork, and stress management supporting academic achievement, social skills, and lifelong health. However, nurturing active lifestyles requires sparking initial interest through options catering to diverse abilities and preferences.

Physical activity provides obvious advantages for children's developing bodies. It builds cardiovascular endurance, muscle strength, and flexibility through activities challenging mobility in playful, curiosity-sparking ways. Sports hone coordination, balance, and proprioception in navigating challenges. They further establish healthy bone density reducing fracture risks and burning calories supporting balanced growth trajectories. Early activity habits also help prevent obesity now impacting youth at alarming rates alongside associated depression, self-image disturbances, and metabolic/immune risks if continued into adulthood.

Movement similarly enhances developing brains and psyches. It reduces stress, anxiety, and depression symptoms through natural mood-improving neurochemical releases like endorphins and dopamine. Sports challenge emotional regulation honing frustration tolerance and cultivating perseverance through practice routines requiring commitment. They foster leadership, independence, and accountability through team and individual positions. Athletic participation boosts self-esteem from physical competence mastery and social connections with peers. Its confidence transfers to academics as concentration, memory, and cognition all benefit from regular exercise in children according to neurological research.

Given exercising's wide-ranging gains, certain approaches motivate youth participation and satisfaction:

Focusing discussions around health, curiosity, and cooperation rather than competition alone lessens performance anxiety as a barrier.

Addressing diverse abilities through multi-level teams, skills workshops or options like yoga, dance, or swimming for cross-training prevents boredom or discouragement.

Parents modeling participation through family activities, attending games, or practicing at home inspire natural enthusiasm.

Drawing connections between practice and incremental skills mastery keeps routines interesting, not frustrating by setting and achieving process-based goals.

Making physical activity inherently social through shared team experiences, games or community clubs enhances appeal and commitment.

Some additional tactics supporting initial enthusiasm for transitioning to lifelong health habits include:

Providing constructive feedback alongside ample praise and high fives keeps children striving purposefully yet carelessly.

Limiting sedentary screen time reallocates more energy towards sports through natural boredom mitigation.

Adjusting schedules allows rest balancing athletic commitments avoiding overuse injuries marring enjoyment.

Tailoring options address individuals' interests through athletics diverse enough keeping novelty while cultivating found passions.

Sparking curiosity around sports sciences' mechanics sustains fascination behind movements and their developing bodies.

Celebrating milestones modestly through family photos, parties or trophies motivates through remembered wins over outlooks on losses.

Ensuring proper diet, rest, and injury prevention through stretching establishes lifetime habits.

Modern society has moved far from ancestral ties to the land, hunting and foraging as life's primary activities shaping human form and function. While technologies confer advantages, disconnecting entirely from nature risks incurring consequences through damaging habits formed from disconnection.

Chief among rising issues stems from nutrition growing increasingly detached from wisdom handed from generation to generation optimizing cellular processes sustaining sentient life across the centuries. However, rekindling ancestral intuition and nurturing balanced nourishment provides an opportunity to regain proprioception diminishing illnesses plaguing overflowing societies. A holistic lifestyle prioritizing both mental acuity and physical sustenance forms the crux of fulfillment across lifetimes.

Ancient cultures intrinsically grasped humanity's full integration within existence's grand scheme, living embedded amid complex webs sustaining all corridors of being. Modern dissociation forgets separation between inner psychology and outer embodiment represents but an illusion, functioning interdependently as yoked partners. Illness arises from disharmonies anywhere along consciousness' profound mind-brain-body continuum damaging the exquisite choreography orchestra conducting trillions of microscopic cellular songbirds melodiously responding to life's arias. Sustaining optimal rhythms demanding synchronization necessitates vigilantly monitoring nourishing impacts rippling outward from decisions pervading tables echoing inward affecting mental rivers feeding spiritual watersheds.

Macro and micronutrients form bricks upon which arise structures supporting supple neural architectures foundational for navigating life's complexities with poise. Deficiencies imperil frameworks through which insight and care emerge while enriching sustenance aids in cultivating virtues serving communities large and small. Vitamins like B and D bolster neurotransmitters relaying electrical impulses guiding steady hands and calm dispositions. Omega-3 fats lubricate synaptic junctions oiling cogs powering focus, memory, and balanced moods. Minerals like magnesium relax tightened muscles and minds alike. Antioxidants flush toxins accumulating amid hassles and protect against cell damage conferring risk for cognitive decline, kept at bay through colorful, antioxidant-dense nourishment. Overall, fuelling disciplined sustenance sustains cognitive powers across generations.

While macronutrients matter, wellness entails more than singular nutrients or prescription regimens alone. An integrated lifestyle nests balanced nourishment amid regular movement, meaningful rest, nurturing relationships, and pursuit of a higher purpose through creativity bringing beauty forth from chaos. Daily activity reconnects one to intrinsic drives animating ancestry inhabiting terrain through cooperation not separation from nature's flowing tapestry. It furthers circulation distributing nutrients throughout whilst flushing toxins accumulated amid stresses natural and imposed. Purposeful movement calms and strengthens in body as within, supported through nourishing diets nourishing cells with primal wisdom cultivating resilience against inevitable adversities life presents all. Together, focus on both nutrition and lifestyle habits bolsters well-being inside and out, anchoring stability and navigating uncertainties.

Adopting holistic nourishment demands commitment but repays abundantly. Centering meals around variety minimizes deficiencies whilst sparking the appetite's curiosity. Emphasize colorful vegetables and fruits in season packing antioxidants; whole grains, nuts, seeds, and legumes fueling steady energy; clean proteins from sustainable sources satiating yet sparing nature's balance. Home cooking nurtures a connection to nourishment's source within balanced schedules preventing burnout. Periodic fasting calms overindulgence's consequences whilst rituals like collective meals strengthen social bonds as ancestors recognized. Movement integrates purposefully yet playfully through activities aligning the body to intrinsic joy. Seeking balance accepts life's uncertainties gracefully whilst nourishment anchors stability amid fluctuating tides. With a dedication to nourishing body matching nourishment within, wellness emerges naturally as life's true purpose springs forth.

Regular activity engenders not only sound bodies but also clear minds, as endorphin release relieves anxieties and depression while aerobic exercise stimulates neurogenesis. Mental diversions accompany physical exertions as cognitive engagement enhances workouts. Yet deeper insights emerge - challenges met fortify perseverance and cultivate optimism that perseverance overcomes all obstacles.

Familiarizing youth with exercise's manifold benefits orients them toward lifelong wellness inherently rewarding. Finding enjoyable activities nurtures intrinsic investment incentivizing continued participation essential to health maintenance. Supportive environments thus constructed carry children aloft on strength and confidence rather than prohibitions alone.

Complementary sustenance completes the developmental regimen, as nutritional adequacy fuels efforts and influences neurochemistry intimately. Mind and metabolism emerge revealed as perpetual dialogue, each impacting the other. Together, balanced fuel and frequent exertions form a robust foundation for indomitable dignity and illuminated potential.

Collectively, these architectures construct lives empowered dynamically to actualize purpose through dedicated care of body and spirit. Resilience shields against tribulations inherent to existence, liberating focus outward to relationships, achievements, and dreams. Suffering loses claims as care of the temple nurtures inhabitant within.

Our investments today herald generations awakened to a partnership where strength, understanding, and hope may flourish for all. Progress bends humanity's arc heavenward as lives are cultivated toward an expression of character's virtues. Such fruits warrant endless cultivation.

Supporting Your Child

The parent-child relationship forms the crucible within which emerges the character capable of shaping society according to either chaos or order through responsible navigation of life's demanding pathways. While external influences impact development, parental ethos instills a foundation upon which arises independence, the care shown towards both self and others and resilience against troubles steering dependable judgment. However, nurturing psychical hardiness necessitates meticulous tending matching affection with accountability empowering the unfolding of virtues across generations.

From earliest utterances signaling dependency's dawning relinquishment, acknowledgment nourishes burgeoning autonomy's roots. Meaningful praise highlighting efforts alongside progress—not innate traits alone—cultivates self-trust guiding explorations beyond comfort's borders. However, validation buttressed by a realistic perspective on strengths awaiting refinement prevents reliance and fosters diligence emerging from within. Feedback channels curiosity towards challenges strengthening competence whilst shielding inexperience from perceived failures inflicting self-doubt. In modeling appreciation of others through affirming words, mirrors form capturing capabilities shining outward to brighten the world.

Alongside independence, intimate bonds prove havens amid life's tempests transforming children into steadfast caretakers. Acceptance of frustrations, sorrows, and joys in full spectra nourishes emotional literacy foundationally bracing against future turbulences. Empathy conveys safe disclosure of all internal tides weathering external stresses, consolidating security allowing vulnerability strengthening intimacy rather than fracturing relationships. Calm mirrors reflection dries tears whilst rain passes, leaving sturdier beaches to weather later storms. Through balanced guidance enabling catharsis besides resilience, sturdy shores rise harboring navigation of ever-changing seas.

Whilst dependence persists, prudent involvement cultivates challenges met creatively without enabling avoidance of difficulties inevitable along maturity's unending road. Brainstorming alternatives before frustration mounts allows perspective recognizing diverse solutions frequently co-exist, empowering ownership of dilemmas emerging from choices rather than blaming elsewhere. Accountability grows through natural responsibilities and consequences facing setbacks without sacrificing self-worth yet retaining optimism from past failures' lessons. Supported experimentation facilitates critical-thinking muscles resolving issues independently yet collaboratively until character forms to weather future adventures.

Foundations require unwavering structure and boundaries aligning conduct befitting a thoughtful role within the community. Consistent routines and reasonable limits instill self-discipline over baseline urges through intrinsic motivation rather than resentment. Appreciating the rationale behind household operations nurtures participation and navigating responsibilities interwoven with privileges. Accepting fairness through open dialogue establishes empathy, integrity, and care beyond oneself rippling into relationships. Respect alongside firmness conveys dignity amid guidance, bolstering independence emerging through choices honoring personal growth and communal welfare.

Child-rearing demands meticulous calibration acknowledging development's pace whilst empowering virtues forming character capable of confronting society's demands. Unconditional validation alongside accountability cultivates self-reliance emerging from inner strength rather than fleeting tropes. Through navigating difficulties reflectively yet supportively, dependability arises in navigating changing social terrain resourcefully. Ultimately, purposeful maturation springs from secure roots within caring communities valuing continual betterment above quick fixes or perceived perfection. With patience and dedication, virtue blooms facing life's uncertainties.

Inner tempests emerge unpredictable yet inevitable, demanding outlets wherein surface. Empathy presents an ear neither passing judgment nor proffering superficial platitudes, but rather reflecting each emotion's embodied truth with presence validating another's full humanity beyond outward appearances. With patience and care, tribulations transform into opportunities fostering resilience against future difficulties through deepened comprehension of alternate viewpoints and life experiences sculpting another. Affirmation restores strength eroded by perils intrinsically navigating existence, whilst shielding vulnerabilities strengthening intimacy rather than jeopardizing rapport.

Alongside comfort, guidance cultivates constructive perseverance in facing life's ongoing uncertainties. Brainstorming diverse approaches and shifting perspectives recognizes multiple strategies coexist in managing difficulties aligned with ethical principles, morality, and future mejor. Modeling patience, integrity, and courage transforms by softening blows life inevitably deals with. Responsiveness nurtures autonomy navigating tribulations reflectively rather than enabling passivity, bolstering empowerment emerging from dedication to continual betterment. Together, empathy and accountability fortify character sustainably confronting society's demands with poise, care, and responsibility.

As dependency diminishes, prudent involvement facilitates challenges overcome through creative, experimental resolutions respecting another's discoveries. Brainstorming options alongside youths grants ownership over issues rather than blaming outwardly, focusing inwardly on efforts and progress rather than fleeting results. Accountability develops through natural duties and consequences faced with emotional regulatory assistance rather than rescuing from experiences inevitably. Supported trial broadens critical thinking and navigates issues autonomously yet interdependently, bolstering self-regulation and reliability upholding relationships, communities, and own well-being upon life's changing courses.

Amid difficulties, gratitude anchors resilience recognizing life's bounties and transcending daily routines. Journaling blessings shifts perspective towards abundance rather than scarcity, fostering perseverance through mindfulness of intrinsic motivations and nourishing self-determination. Together, empathy, validation, and accountability fortify character sustainably facing tomorrow's uncertainties with generosity, care, and humility. Ultimately, nurturance cultivates dependability navigating existence's fluctuations resourcefully yet cooperatively, standing resolute yet malleable amid life's perpetual unfolding.

Most fundamentally, availability conveys another's worthiness of dedicated vigor in navigating life's obstacles. Quality interactions nurture secure roots reinforcing dignity amid struggles, whereas fleeting contact risks instilling transitory significance condoned by distraction. Modeling engaged listening without judgment and affirming intrinsic virtues fosters initiative emerging from inner strength rather than momentary pleasures. Belonging emerges from stability amid flux, as adaptation forms to society's shifting tides bolstered by community-prioritizing relationships sustaining global civilization's advance.

Early relations forge a character's blueprint, as formative interactions entrench secure bases permitting later experimentation. Consistent compassion molds relational trust catalyzing burgeoning autonomy from the root outwardly. Quality interactions enlighten worth far surpassing fleeting achievements, modeling conscientious livelihoods navigating lifelong difficulties cooperatively. Engrossment instills belonging's depth stabilizing against future solitude whilst appreciating another's intrinsic dignity unconditionally. Together, belonging and accountability cultivate independence emerging from internal strength and facing society honorably.

Meaningful involvement sparks curiosity navigating developing interests deftly.

Attentiveness elevates endeavors nourishing emerging motivations, as perseverance arises naturally pursuing unified aspirations. Providing guidance rather than direction respects unfolding autonomy, embracing mistakes as learning irrespective of results. Shared dedication cultivates responsibility recognizing impacts upon familial welfare and community threads sustaining civilization. Purpose emerges through cooperative betterment witnessed daily, motivating resilience amid inevitable hindrances.

Moreover, participation supports character maturing adaptively. Exposure diversifies comprehension bolstering flexible navigation unforeseeable interruptions. Dialogues model empathy, integrity, and reliability easing inevitable perturbations. Appreciation anchors pride from intrinsic virtues exceeding status. Responsiveness elevates problem-solving emerging from dedication to relationships surmounting obstacles resourcefully. Authenticity conveys another's worth far surpassing outward productivity, cultivating generosity despite changing seasons. Engrossment sustains dignity facing tomorrow confidently yet collaboratively.

As growing independence necessitates stumbles, safety nets provide ballast without enabling passivity. Availability conveys dedication towards continual enrichment beyond momentary pleasures. Challenges emerge creatively tackled through cooperation respecting another's discoveries.

Accountability emerges from natural duties with emotional regulatory support rather than absolving from valuable lessons. Supported trials broaden adaptive, critical thinking navigating issues autonomously amid community. Ultimately, presence affirms another's significance beyond shifting circumstances whilst empowering self-reliance.

Supportive presence throughout development's journey constructs an environmental bastion of security and belief within which character may bloom unfettered. Empathetic validation of experiences lived, however trivial externally, nourishes introspection enabling perspective maturation. Comfort nourishes courage to encounter complexities sure to arise, liberating focus outward to relationships and purpose.

Bonding cultivated through quality engagement anchors this foundation of strength, as empathy, encouragement, and patience speaks volumes exceeding surfaces. Dialogue and shared interest nurture understanding exceeding external incentives, empowering autonomy and identity rooted in virtue rather than fleeting reward dynamics. Resolve emerges fortified where vulnerability once thrived.

Together, these developmental currents orient lives intrinsically toward purposeful participation and equity, unfettered by circumstances transient in the grandest view.

Challenges greet not as obstacles circumscribing potential, but adventures wherein perseverance overcomes all impediments and relationship enriches common pursuits of dignity. Suffering loses claim where the temple's inhabitants emerge thus nurtured.

Progress bends its arc heavenward as generations inherit strengths cultivated with compassion. Our investment, however small, portends societies awakened to a partnership where understanding, courage, and creativity may flourish unrestrained. In such equitable sharing, humankind's fullest blossoming comes into focus.

Challenges and Setbacks

While cultivating strong qualities of self-discipline and boundaries is crucial for personal and professional advancement, establishing these traits often faces considerable hurdles. Whether stemming from internal or external forces, impediments to disciplined behavior can undermine even the most well-intentioned goals and ambitions if left unrecognized and unchecked. However, through self-reflection and a commitment to continuous betterment, individuals possess the capacity to surmount typical barriers and foster the discipline necessary for thriving.

One of the most pervasive obstacles worldwide is procrastination - the habitual delay of tasks and responsibilities despite acknowledging their importance. Neurological research indicates procrastination arises from an imbalanced interaction between the prefrontal cortex region governing self-control and the part of the brain triggering reward responses. As immediate gratification takes precedence over long-term goals, important duties are neglected in favor of more enticing yet less productive activities.

While procrastination may provide momentary relief or distraction, its consequences become increasingly detrimental over time. Missing deadlines, committing sub-par work, and accruing stress from lingering obligations corrode self-confidence and undermine life satisfaction. Furthermore, habitual procrastination fosters a cycle of avoidance wherein tasks grow more formidable due to their prolongation, necessitating even greater willpower to initiate.

However, procrastination need not define nor dictate one's ability to follow through on commitments. The first step is attaining clarity on precisely when why, and how delaying tendencies typically manifest. Do obligations linger until the eleventh hour? Is preparation postponed for more appealing pastimes?

Answering such questions builds self-awareness of personal triggers.

From there, systematic changes can be implemented to disrupt procrastinatory routines. Breaking large undertakings into smaller, more manageable tasks reduces their perceived daunting nature. Setting tight, non-negotiable deadlines with accountability partners also helps stay on track. Recognizing that feelings of anxiety or resistance are normal parts of any difficult job can empower continued forward motion despite inner protestations. With consistency, new disciplined patterns of early preparation and diligent follow-through can replace delayed reactions as habitual responses.

Another pervasive impediment is fluctuating levels of motivation that stem from an absence of clearly defined values or objectives. Without a compelling reason or vision pulling one forward, maintaining self-discipline proves challenging as drive wanes. However, lack of inspiration often originates from an unreflective life drifting along pre-set societal conventions rather than one firmly rooted in personal meaning.

Taking time for deep introspection to uncover core interests, talents, and priorities provides internal fuel when external forces tempt diluting dedication. Writing down life purpose and values in a personal mission statement gives concrete direction to stay motivated, even through difficulties or distractions.

Additionally, surrounding oneself with like-minded individuals pursuing purposeful work creates a supportive, inspirational atmosphere for continued growth.

Because inspiration is sometimes elusive, proactively taking small, regular steps toward important objectives also nourishes intrinsic motivation over the long run through a sense of progress. Agreed-upon accountability with others involved in similar pursuits prevents wavering commitment. Reframing demanding tasks as investments in one's development counters thoughts of mundanity to spark passion anew. With applied effort, inspiration springs less from fleeting whims and more from consciously cultivating purpose and meaning in all endeavors.

Living in an era emphasizing the pursuit of pleasure and leisure presents a significant challenge for developing self-discipline, as immersive digital technologies and social media actively pull focus from responsibilities. Constant notifications, updates, and alerts trigger reward responses that diminish willpower reserves. Furthermore, comparisons to highlight reels of others' lavish lifestyles on social media can foster envious cravings for luxury and promote perceptions that discipline denies enjoyment.

However, maintaining discipline does not preclude enjoyment - it simply entails delaying some immediate thrills for greater long-term fulfillment. Setting aside devices for blocks of focused productivity prevents distraction, and curating social media to avoid envy-inducing comparisons supports focus on personal goals. It is also wise to reflect on whether perceived friends primarily encourage leisure over diligence, and consider limiting exposure to such influences if they regularly undermine dedication.

Ultimately, cultivating self-discipline involves selectively blocking external forces pushing instant gratification so internal motivations for holistic well-being and deeper satisfaction can instead steer behavior. With practice, discomfort can be experienced by such forces, and pleasure derived from steady progress toward important objectives rather than fleeting pleasures denying fulfillment.

Strong willpower emerges from the courage to deliberately unplug some indulgences society deems mandatory.

Common impediments like habitual procrastination, lack of motivation, and social pressures toward instant gratification cannot be shrugged off but must be directly confronted through awareness, planning, and perseverance. The initial step is honestly assessing internal and external influences typically undermining discipline without judgment.

From there, a systematic approach focusing on manageable behavior changes establishes new routines overriding autopilot responses. Crucially, remaining non-punitive and celebrating each instance of strengthened willpower sustains long-term transformation. With a dedication to continual betterment, self-discipline arises not as a fleeting state but as a cultivated trait supporting personal growth regardless of surrounding conditions.

One of the most effective means of confronting motivational lulls or hesitation stems from establishing unambiguous, measurable objectives. Clear goals confer direction and closure to tasks, while their attainment bolsters self-efficacy and sustains passion. Specific, moderately sized targets set shortly also help maintain momentum by dividing large aims into bite-sized stages conducive to continuous progress.

Ideally, goals should be:

Personally meaningful - Intrinsic to values, priorities, interests
Challenging yet realistic - Stretch current abilities somewhat
Specific and quantified - e.g. "write 1,000 words daily" not "be productive"
Time-bound - Include clear deadlines to stay accountable

Writing goals down makes them tangible, while visually posting reminders keeps them consciously top-of-mind. Reviewing and revising aims periodically adapts them to changing circumstances or lessons learned.

Additionally, breaking work into timed, focused sessions using the Pomodoro Technique (25 minutes work, 5 minutes break) concentrates attention for optimal productivity and avoids languishing between tasks. Regular reflection on accomplishments fueled by the satisfaction of checking off-targets in planners or apps also bolsters perseverance.

Alongside purposeful objectives, efficient time management through prioritization is essential to avoid procrastination and wasted hours. However, prioritization requires discerning between urgent pressing issues and important long-term priorities - often conflated amid the daily bustle.

Some suggestions include:

Scheduling protected blocks for high-yield activities

Batching similar tasks to minimize context-switching

Delegating lower-value duties to free up discretionary time

Limiting distraction-prone locations/devices during focus periods

Monthly/weekly planning to envision upcoming responsibilities

Saying "no" to some discretionary commitments if over-scheduled

Using a calendar makes scheduling tangible obligations effortless. Listing all daily tasks by priority alongside estimated durations also provides clarity on how to maximize productivity during available periods. Regularly reviewing schedules prevents last-minute rushing and the attendant suboptimal work quality or missed deadlines.

At their core, daily habits powerfully shape behaviors and the paths lives ultimately follow. Developing supportive habits is key to overcoming recurring hurdles through automatizing discipline until virtue becomes second nature. Successful creation of new habits relies upon:

Isolating a specific, measurable behavior - e.g. morning exercise
Establishing clear cues/triggers for when the behavior occurs - e.g. after breakfast

Maximizing rewards and positive reinforcement of new routine

Some disciplined habits to consider include morning routines for focused starts, dedicated study/work areas devoid of distractions, regular exercise/nutrition schedules, and consistent bedtime routines supporting rest and recharge. Habit-tracking apps provide satisfaction from visual progress markers that sustain routines. Overall, small deliberate adjustments create compounding long-term impacts.

Sustainable change inherently involves accountability to curtail sole reliance on willpower susceptible to fluctuation. Structured support systems rally motivation during lulls by offering nonjudgmental guidance, advice, and incentives to adhere to goals through participative communities.

While private accountability partners judiciously review plans and successes, public commitment amplifies resolve. Joining online groups, challenges, or coworking spaces for mutual motivation keeps isolated individuals on track through social proof of others' diligence.

Inspiring mentors also aid by modeling discipline and validating temporary setbacks as normal rather than shortcomings requiring perfectionism. Overall, healthy communities reinforce discipline as an admirable trait uplifting all members rather than a lonely battle. Interdependence strengthens perseverance when autonomy poses risks of reconsideration during difficulties.

Maintaining self-discipline involves an endless refining process as inevitable setbacks will occur requiring adaptation and renewed diligence. Persistence lies in accepting discipline as a work-in-progress strengthened daily rather than an unattainable perfect state. Grace and understanding toward inevitable mistakes prevent harsh self-criticism from undermining progress.

Viewing discipline as an exciting challenge empowering personal evolution rather than a chore boosts perseverance. Overall, a growth mindset acknowledges discipline as a continually cultivated asset through ever-deepening self-awareness and targeted strategies. Approaching obstacles methodically with patience and community support ultimately fosters an empowering and self-sustaining discipline.

From withstanding brief discomforts to achieving new milestones, to dealing composedly with social difficulties or academic frustrations, the ability to patiently endure is profoundly beneficial to a child's balanced development. Numerous studies show developing patience correlates with lower stress levels, superior coping mechanisms, higher achievement, and stronger relationships as youth mature into adulthood.

Patience aids learning by tolerating setbacks inevitable in any skill acquisition. The steadfast who persevere despite initial failures tend to integrate new abilities more thoroughly with experience. Similarly, cultivating composure aids in forming friendships by suspending rash reactions and considering others' perspectives in conflicts.

Patience even buoys physical health. Those who can delay gratification exhibit healthier lifestyle habits, report less illness, and recover at a swifter pace - likely due to reduced stress chemicals emitted during impatience. Far from restrictive, patience thus allows children to fully reap the rewards of efforts by forestalling impulsiveness impeding clear focus and outcomes.

As any parent knows, instilling virtues takes consistent modeling more than strict commanding. Children inherently imitate how adults handle boredom, frustration, or delayed results. Remaining composed through minor irritations and viewing difficulties as natural, temporary, and able to be overcome through steady effort, sets the paramount example.

Focusing on process over product also inspires perseverance. Discussing strategies, progress made and insights learned from challenges maintains momentum, versus praising only end achievements. Specifically acknowledging and rewarding instances of patience, such as sticking with instrumental practice or difficult puzzles, reinforces the behavior.

Simultaneously, parents must carefully consider a child's individual needs, abilities, and interests to set reasonable expectations. An overly rigid "just keep trying" mantra may backfire by discouraging risk-taking essential for learning. Implementing variations, creative breaks, or scaling back overwhelming tasks fosters perseverance through success and sustained motivation versus coerced obedience. Striking this balance builds confidence in one's capacities.

How parents frame instances of impatience, frustration, or failure when they inevitably occur also influences a child's relationship with adversity. While natural emotions should never be suppressed, they can be reframed through a perspective focused on growth instead of outcomes.

Discussing setbacks as common, valuable parts of progress prepares children to view mistakes or delays gracefully versus cataclysms. Affirming efforts and positive attitudes amid missteps bolsters resilience to rebound steadily. With guidance, children learn regarding difficulties hopefully despite the present disappointment, knowing new insights will emerge from reflection on experiences.

Rather than resentment toward those excelling with apparent ease, patience embraces diverse paths and talents, realizing natural variations exist and one's worth derives from diligent effort regardless. This gratitude perspective nurtures compassion to encourage others to persevere. Overall, patience imbues challenges with fulfillment through Wisdom gleaned, relationships deepened and strengths realized - far outweighing fleeting pleasures or addictions to haste and hype.

Integrating relaxing pastimes into a schedule helps develop the composure essential for patience. Free explorations ignite curiosity and relieve pent frustrations, whether through artistic expression, hands-on tinkering, outdoor play in nature, or other personally meaningful activities. These provide perspective-widening breaks during or after difficult periods to recharge.

Additionally, practicing calming techniques like deep breathing, meditation, yoga, or journaling during childhood makes managing stressors second nature. Implemented judiciously amidst youthful energies, such methods enhance clarity and focus, preserving patience amid distractions. Overall, fostering an environment that continually nurtures well-being through a balance of challenges and rest equips children internally to persist with poise.

While impatience panders to the allure of immediacy, patience proves itself in the quiet accomplishments of steadfast endurance. Through cultivating this virtue amidst today's distractions, a lifelong resilience forms enabling children to achieve unhindered. Far from a loss, delayed pleasures are gained through deepened understanding, wisdom, and personal growth born of facing obstacles with sustained conviction. Ultimately, the reward of patience lies in empowering children to thrive according to their schedule and vision regardless of society's clamors for instant gratification.

Self-discipline emerges not through fleeting prohibitions alone, but through dedicated appreciation of priorities warranted by dreams and relationships. Procrastination loses power whereas discipline arises intrinsically from vigilant self-awareness and goal-actualization. Boundaries thus anchored nourish autonomy unfettered by external circumstances.

Addressing inevitable challenges demands not reaction but perspective - patience permits wisdom from mistakes however frustrating initially. Support networks strengthen where vulnerability once reigned. Resolutions borne of introspection carry farther than mandates externally imposed.

Children learn trials mark not failure but preparation for success sure to follow, in time's fullness, if resolve persists. Optimism supplants resignation where impatience once inflamed, empowering character-driven lives of purpose, creativity, and dignity.

Together these developmental bastions fortify against complexity's natural unevenness, liberating focus to relationships, achievements, and dreams. Resilience emerges less as a consequence than choice - a choice nurtured within through confidence that small steps lead inexorably to great heights if patience guides the way.

Our shared work today nourishes not only youth but the world increasingly recognizing shared stake in each other's welfare and rights. Progress bends its arc heavenward as strengths cultivated here ripple outward on time's stream, touching an ever-expanding circus with hope reborn. Such gifts warrant cultivation till Earth's final sunset.

Age-Specific Strategies

Providing optimum support for a child's development relies upon comprehending their evolving capacities and proclivities at each stage. However, societal conventions or personal agendas can distort realistic impressions of a young person's readiness, undermining the nurturing relationship essential to maturation.

Establishing reasonable expectations starts with gaining perspective on typical developmental sequences. Major strides in cognitive, emotional, and social domains tend to emerge sequentially according to neurobiological preparedness over infancy, childhood, and youth.

While variations exist, general milestones provide context. For example, the egocentrism of early years yields to acknowledging others' vantage points by school age with appropriate modeling. Meanwhile, a toddler's limited vocabulary precludes intricate explanations their growing prefrontal cortex will shortly handle.

Proactively recognizing present competencies avoids either under- or overestimating a child. This spares them undue stress or boredom and promotes a resilient sense of capability.

Dialogue geared appropriately to challenges without overwhelming.

Beyond aggregate developmental patterns, each child's intrinsic tendencies also affect how guidance lands. More sensitive natures may require calmer instruction than spirited peers. Those cautiously processing changes benefit patience rather than haste.

Attentively understanding inclinations like preferred learning styles, sensitivity levels, and innate risk-taking comfort zones aids sensitively designing the optimal scaffolding. Allowing preferred outlets for communicating needs, within reason, cultivates cooperation.

Affirming individual strengths amid areas requiring finesse bolsters confidence essential for experimenting outside comfort zones. Still, pushing comfort boundaries too ambitiously risks damaging trust in the relationship. Gradualness and compromise optimize learning climates.

Judiciously graduated challenges inspire striving while cementing belief in one's capabilities. Starting initiatives manageable yet novel prevents frustration and exhausting motivation. Graciously acknowledging attempts preserves enthusiasm for refining skills.

Conversely, prolonging support for past independence invites co-dependency.

Watchfully supporting budding autonomy with safety nets for stumbles respects burgeoning decision-making. Offering guidance primarily regarding processes and strategies, versus automatic solutions, nurtures problem-solving muscle.

Regular reassessments adapt latitude to expanding competencies. Reflecting on the perspective gained from both mistakes and triumphs sustains progress by continually recalibrating the balance between respite and rigor according to changing needs.

Honest yet compassionate communication about performance clarifies while bolstering willpower. Specifically addressing conduct or domains requiring adaptation preserves dignity far beyond vague criticism. Expressing assured belief in abilities to reform fortifies motivation to refine.

Inviting open discussion on perceptions and goals invites partnership for change from shared understanding versus dictated obedience. Nonjudgmentally exploring emotional roots of behaviors insights resolutions respecting individuality.

With time, as trust endures, even difficult conversations strengthen relationships by proving commitment to maximizing potential rather than control. And as abilities burgeon, so too should involvement in setting expectations to internalize responsibility and self-direction.

Striking this balance between high expectations and empathy satisfies basic human needs for both challenge and support essential to thriving. Through attentiveness, adjustment, and caring dialogue, guidance is nurtured from wherever children stand rather than ideals disconnected from realities. In this spirit, individuals best self-actualize according to their own distinctive pace and character.

The tumultuous toddler years introduce children to life's endless possibilities alongside boundaries maintaining balance. During intensifying curiosity, discipline provides structure permitting safer discovery. Yet rigidness thwarts the spirited self-asserting necessary for independence. This epoch thus demands steadiness and flexibility.

At this stage, structure arises less from abstract ethics than concrete habits securing basic comforts. Consistency begins through a limited lexicon describing needs, like kindness, sharing, and eating schedules. Visual cues or signals supplement limited vocabularies. Predictability relieves anxieties accompanying overwhelming independence. Rules convey care through reliable rhythms amid flux. Repetition alleviates relying upon impulse alone. And gradual exposures to larger worlds cultivate comfort beyond thresholds.

Consequences logically follow transgressions proportionate to the intent's absence at this age. Removals redirect energy constructively rather than punish. Calm explanations reconnect missteps to solutions strengthening resolve for future success and connection with caregivers. Rules simply state rather than reason prematurely for still-forming logic. Trust proceeds obedience until rationales develop comprehending rules' design for group wellbeing. For now, judicious boundaries liberate focus onto growth itself.

At every opportunity, successes receive acknowledgment inspiring persistence when difficulties arrive. Yet praise emphasizes observed qualities - like sharing toys or using words for needs - avoiding hollow platitudes.

Catching positive behaviors maintains eagerness to please as logic develops grasping complex interactions. Smiles, high-fives, or a fun activity together rewards efforts for emulation.

Requests utilize compassionate yet expectant tones subtly encouraging cooperation. Redirecting through modeled alternatives introduces improved options organically. And breaks for play rebuild will be taxed by new habits, recharging motivation for further progress. This balance avoids coercing assent before volition grows. Instead, consistent affection and constructive incentives internalize principles as innate sensibilities guiding preferences naturally with maturity. Order emerges freely within compassion.

Repetition secures young psyches to adapt beyond initial dependencies. Meal, sleep, and activity routines become calendars making once-foreign habits comfortably predictable.

Sameness permits concentration on enrichment like reading or play rather than uncertainty. Yet flexibility maintains spontaneity vitalizing routines. Occasional alterations introduce adaptability crucial for resilience when change inevitably comes.

Preparation minimizes unpredictability by signaling imminent transitions. Timers visualize waiting periods's ends. Step-by-step walkthroughs of unfamiliar processes give handholds for nervous stability.

Overall rhythms balance stimulating discovery and restorative continuity. In this climate self-possession forms, empowering expanding spheres of mastery and joyous engagement with life in all its fullness. Order arises from balance itself. Establishing this equilibrium demands vigilance, patience, and care. But seeds sown here take root as characteristics of strength, integrity, and love sustain lives throughout their unfoldment. In guidance resides humanity's hope.

The elementary years inaugurate intellects into realms begging discovery. As logic blooms, responsibility expands, yet freedom remains new. This period thus necessitates optimizing independence within prudent boundaries. Rules clarify duties as privileges grow. Lessons cultivate potential through playful yet earnest activities.

Mistakes introduce lessons versus condemnation at this sensitive stage. And steadfast role models demonstrate pathways traversing life's obstacles honorably. In nurturing wonder and fortitude equally, youngsters claim authority guiding their growth bravely into maturity.

At this age, dependence transitions to cooperation with guidance. Rules articulate expectations now understood through reason rather than just obedience.

Children's emerging problem-solving aids shared agreements beneficial to all. Chores promote dignity through contributions. And considering consequences before acting encourages deliberation over impulse.

Mistakes elicit conversations examining why and how to improve, avoiding shame undermining motivation. Praise highlights diligence itself over actions, instilling habits in the industry.

Gradual release of duties as abilities emerge respects growing autonomy. Successes feel self-driven rather than rewarded for compliance. In responsibility resides purpose and care for others' well-being.

The play remains crucial at any age for exploring potential. Yet focused, goal-directed games also impart applicable skills. Roleplaying daily routines or hypothetical scenarios rehearses complex interactions. Structured projects integrate core learning into enthusiastic creations. Competitions introduce cooperation and healthy frustration.

Practice builds mastery through perseverance essential for any undertaking. Yet continual enjoyment prevents boredom from hampering progress. Achievable challenges but frequent encouragement sustains gusto where defeats may discourage.

Overall a disposition takes shape through simulation - of managing feelings, navigating social dynamics, and directing energies productively even under stress or disappointment. Confidence forms through the character itself.

Early interests indicate potential needing fostering. Discussions connect interests and schoolwork to life's richness. Yet guidance respects wonder as its reward over mere utility. Questions elicit patient, truthful answers satisfying innate searches for meaning without depriving discoveries. Resource lists substitute for direct answers permitting independent research.

Budding creativity flourishes through experimentation with supportive guidance. Setbacks pose opportunities to consider alternate routes through life's obstacles. Joy arises from personal engagement and resilience itself.

This latitude within caring parameters and honest counsel cultivates self-directed thinkers equipped to transform what they encounter through perseverance and compassion. Equipped thus, all roads lead toward a life lived fully. Fostering these proclivities responsibly navigates formative years. Young pioneers emerge filled with purpose, strength and care for fellow travelers along humanity's path. Greater gifts no phase of life can confer.

Adolescence initiates a profound metamorphosis demanding sage yet non-intrusive care. As physical and intellectual changes arouse new sensibilities and proclivities, ancient precedents provide ballast amid turbulent emerging independence. This precarious passage necessitates trust balanced by concern. While authority relinquishes direct domination, counsel remains available without judgment, empowering youths' expanding stewardship. Mistakes pose opportunities to strengthen resolve rather than regret.

Overall rhythms adjust according to nature's unfolding design. For now, environments accommodate flux; later reflection illuminates deeper purposes. If guided thus with empathy and wisdom, today's uncertainty cultivates tomorrow's stewardship.

At this crossroads, boundaries clarify without constraining burgeoning autonomy. Rules reflect mutual care and consequence rather than control.

Limits curb impulses endangering wellbeing and future options. Yet room remains to safely express emerging identities and preferences. Requirements promote responsibility instead of reactionism.

Consequences logically relate to actions and youths' increasing capacity for deliberation. Still, clemency acknowledges development's sensitivity. Overall trust and consistent enforcement foster the integrity necessary to navigate life's complexity.

Advisors model principled reasoning over absolute dictates. Open discussions uncover the rationale for cultivating vision beyond present restrictions. Compromise respects maturing judgment guiding decisions gradually to self-sufficiency.

Boundaries permit focusing outward and establishing inner authority essential for life's unfolding journey. Order arises within freedom.

Adolescence instigates innate desires to contribute and belong amid life's mysteries.

Guidance supports quests aligning talents and passions for meaningful engagement.

Exposure to disciplines, philosophies, and roles in navigating life's challenges empowers the recognition of aligned paths. Mentors demonstrate perseverance wherever interests take root.

Yet authority also respects privacy for autonomous investigation and discovery. Questions elicit wisdom cultivating independent worldviews. Critiques focus on reasoning not identities.

Overall an environment provides anchorage as youths' capacities expand. Within security, curiosity flourishes, cultivating identities and directing changes rather than surrendering to them. Emerging purpose arises from within.

Adulthood initiates accountability demanding progressive preparation. Responsible freedoms teach managing limitations before fully testing them.

Simulated consequences through transparent discussion of everyday dilemmas enlighten without endangering. Problem-solving skills nurtured now meet future obstacles with poise.

Guidance remains available without directing lives, respecting hard-earned perspective. Plans receive consideration and reality-checks mitigating pessimism and naivety.

Compassion reflects recognizable emotions, redeeming potential within inevitable missteps. Mistakes cultivate resilience greater than flawless compliance.

In balance encouragement and prudence accompany youths' maturation. Life's mysteries and hard-won stability equip emerging stewardship for humanity's future and goodness' unending unfolding.

Age-appropriate strategies prove essential, as receptive capacities, motivations, and challenges shift predictably across life's unfolding seasons. Tailoring expectations, language, and involvements to unique requisites nurtures progression optimized according to phase and circumstance. Reaction gives way to comprehension as roles adapt collaboratively.

Guidance of the youngest minds emphasizes security, exploration, and virtue's lessons conveyed simply through repetitions, boundaries, and praise. Independence buds where dependencies once reigned. Formative skills thus imprinted continue bearing fruit into maturity.

School-aged years cultivate emergent capabilities and identities, as problem-solving, accountability, and compassion cultivate strength beyond early dependencies. Creativity flourishes where rules once constrained potential. Responsibility emerges less as a duty than opportunity and adventure.

Adolescence demands sympathetic navigations anew, as autonomy, purpose, and integrity claims supersede childhood's protections. Perspective, not prohibition, proves ally as life roles expand. Relationships shift from directive to collaborative, carrying youths aloft on empowerment and care.

Coordinated developmental architectures emerge, empowering lives unfettered by circumstance to actualize dignity through character over time. Challenges greet not as impediments, but as opportunities to strengthen resolve and relationships in partnership. Progress continues bending its arc heavenward as strengths thus cultivating uplift not only individuals but worlds increasingly inclined to equity, compassion, and shared welfare in our global village. Such gifts warrant perpetual cultivation.

Digital Age

Advancements in digital technologies over the past couple of decades have radically transformed the way we live, work, and interact with one another. Once purely physical, our world has become increasingly virtual as well—augmented by devices, screens, algorithms, and online networks that connect us across space and time. For young people today growing up immersed in this digital world, it can be difficult to discern where the real ends and the virtual begins.

While technology undoubtedly enriches our lives in countless ways, it would be irresponsible not to also consider its potential shadow sides and unintended consequences—especially concerning developing minds that are still learning how to navigate reality. Children are among the most avid users and adopters of new technologies, yet their youthful sensitivity leaves them particularly vulnerable to certain risks in unsupervised virtual spaces. With social media and the internet now effectively ubiquitous, an undeniable impact on mental health and well-being has emerged that warrants close discussion and mitigation through responsible parenting.

Constant connectivity is perhaps the defining feature of life online today. Smartphones in particular have facilitated an "always on" relationship with virtual networks that know few bounds of time or place. But constant access to dopamine-inducing notifications, updates, and virtual reward systems comes at a cost. For developing young minds, the lure of perpetual stimulation risks crowding out opportunities for solitude, contemplation, and real-world socialization—all formative experiences that enhance self-awareness, resilience, and interpersonal skills.

Time spent immersed in virtual reality competes directly with activities required for healthy psychosocial development, like face-to-face social interactions, physical exercise, creative hobbies, and simply perceiving the world with undivided attention. Numerous studies suggest problematic internet use is positively correlated with depression, anxiety, loneliness, and even symptoms of obsessive-compulsive disorder among children and teenagers. Overreliance on technology-mediated communication may limit the formation of satisfying social bonds and skills like reading non-verbal facial cues—crucial not only for peer relationships but for navigating everyday life offline as well.

One underlying issue appears to be how constant connectivity disincentivizes mental "downtime" required for rest and recovery. The unending scroll of social updates and notifications overrides our brain's innate abilities to filter out distractions and selectively attend to what is most pertinent, important, or worthwhile. As cognitive resources are increasingly committed to virtual rather than physical realities, abilities like concentration, reflection, and self-directed deep thinking suffer. This constant distraction further breeds anxiety—as youth internalize an always-on availability that is ultimately unsustainable, yet feel compelled to participate out of fear of missing out.

The inescapable presence of peers just a click or tap away can also exacerbate insecurities through unfavorable social comparisons. Envy emerges as highlight reels of others' lives are endlessly consumed, while the inevitable imperfections of real relationships fade into the backdrop. Even the most well-adjusted young people may find their self-esteem fluctuations tethered to arbitrary "likes" and comments populated by fleeting viral content rather than substantive connection. Over time, the resulting bruised self-image risks morphing anxiety into full-blown depression if left to fester without intervention.

Decreased face-to-face interactions and meaningful social ties in turn feed into feelings of loneliness, despite seeming "connected" at all times. Constant connectivity becomes paradoxical isolation, as the most intimate human needs for meaningful presence, compassion, and shared experiences with real people in physical co-presence go unmet. This discordance threatens not only mental health, but the very capacity to forge deep relationships so essential for individual growth and well-being across the lifespan. No algorithm or virtual system can replace these fundamental human requirements, so addressing the imbalance is an urgent societal concern.

To safeguard children's well-being amid these challenging societal shifts, conscientious parenting and guidance must thoughtfully address new forms of risk while embracing opportunities. Open communication, trusting relationships, and leadership through positive example can effectively steer youth away from potential pitfalls, towards developing resilience and responsibility regarding their technology use. With care and wisdom, guardians can help the next generation thoughtfully integrate useful virtual tools into lives still rooted primarily in reality—not withdraw into isolation or extremism, but learn to navigate both physical and digital worlds.

Establishing clear rules, routines, and monitoring provides the structure that maintains children's safety and priorities online. Setting age-appropriate limits regarding screen time, applications permitted, and account privacy settings reduces overexposure to risqué content or unrestricted contact with strangers. Periodic family discussions keep lines of understanding open to address issues proactively rather than reactively— empowering youth to make safe, thoughtful choices aligned with their growth into independent and compassionate individuals.

Parents and caregivers must also lead by positive example, modeling balanced technology habits of their own. Phones down during mealtimes, limited usage before bed, and device-free vacations demonstrate how virtual connectivity enhances rather than controls daily life. Prioritizing face-to-face family time, outdoor activities and creative hobbies gives children alternatives to fill any latent anxiety around device deprivation, replacing compulsive scrolling with meaningful experiences. In this way, responsibility regarding technology becomes a collaborative effort of guardianship—not authoritarian restrictions, but open-hearted guidance empowering youth to find their appropriate rhythms of online and offline lives.

Shaping a thoughtful relationship with virtual tools early on has enduring benefits. It cultivates resilience when inevitable distractions or even unhealthy peer influences arise down the line. Youth who value in-person interactions over virtual approval are less vulnerable to problematic internet use. Those comfortable with solitude can better manage comparisons online without threat to self-worth. Most importantly, prioritizing real human relationships protects against the paradoxical isolation that leaves constant connectivity a more sedentary shell than the fulfillment of innate connection-seeking. Approached wisely as partners in guidance, conscientious parenting can help the next generation thoughtfully reap technology's benefits while avoiding its potential costs to well-being.

Establishing consistent rules around how much and what kind of screen engagement is allowed establishes a structure crucial to responsibility. Regular break points prevent compulsive use from crowding out other priorities, from physical activity to social interaction to schoolwork, art, and play. Strict time limits matched to age and maturity reduce susceptibility to infinite online distraction. Guidelines clarify reasonable exceptions for projects versus casual use, balancing flexibility with consistency. Shared family devices in common areas also facilitate parental monitoring versus isolating engagement behind closed doors. While digital natives are themselves learning balance, setting compassionate yet firm boundaries supports focus on holistic wellness over compulsive scrolling and gaming alone.

The examples parents set through their technology habits speak volumes in imparting wisdom to impressionable youth. When mealtimes prioritize presence over phones, bedtimes remain device-free zones, and family vacations disconnected, consistency models balanced use without depriving digital benefits altogether. It teaches respecting others' attention and time instead of constant online compulsions. Responsible leadership considers not only time dedicated to screening oneself, but quality of content—prioritizing education, creativity, community, and mental enrichment over mindless consumption. By demonstrating discipline, discernment, and digital citizenship through actions, households nurture the same in their children at a formative developmental stage.

Establishing basic controls like restricted search functions, privacy settings, and age-appropriate access directly safeguards youth from potential dangers online such as exposure to inappropriate images or private contact with strangers. It communicates respect and protection of innocence without implicit distrust. Open communication allows clarifying any confusion constructively instead of reactively—whether discussing concerns personally or utilizing parental monitoring and reporting tools, the intent remains guidance not restriction. Accountability in all directions fosters the understanding that technology, though offering opportunity, requires ongoing education in navigating thoughtfully and safely. Households stay aware of evolving issues to keep children protected without unduly limiting natural curiosity or the potential for good online either.

Rather than authoritarian rules alone, open communication allows for addressing concerns proactively through understanding. It invites youth to bring challenges to trusted counsel freely without fear of reprimand. Regular check-ins keep parental awareness calibrated to children's changing interests and activities online. In turn, transparency fosters accountability—encouraging responsibility regarding content shared, the privacy of personal information, and discerning safe from harmful influences. With guidance in navigating complex online social worlds thoughtfully, youth feel empowered to handle minor issues independently while recognizing wisdom in experience to seek help in uncertain situations too. Empathy, trust, and collaboration replace reactivity to cultivate patience, judgment, and resilience through partnership rather than conflict.

While reasonable limits secure well-being, prohibition teaches nothing but rebellion. Families integrate technology advantageously by suggesting constructive creative, social, and learning applications—setting an example of innovative and enriching use. Shared discovery of educational tools nurtures interests and skills, from coding to photography, writing to music. Facilitating participation in online communities of shared passions replaces the dangers of aimless wandering. Limiting casual use opens bandwidth for deeper cyber connections and projects alongside real-world socializing and activities. Balance considers technology an enhancement, not a replacement for well-rounded growth—a supplementary rather than defining element of children's lives.

Even with proactive guidance, lapses may still occur as digital natives learn self-regulation.

Empathy and understanding recognize youthful judgment develops gradually through experience, not perfection. Temporary and thoughtful consequences, combined with open discussion reinforcing care, wisdom, and accountability, cultivate humility and maturation far better than harsh reactions that fail to teach. With rule-breaks addressed privately and respectfully, suspicion gives way to trust allowing honest disclosure of issues early for resolution. Discernment also considers severity and intent versus zero-tolerance, balancing discretion with accountability. Ultimately, a compassionate home focused on education over enforcement nurtures responsible citizenship through cooperation rather than fear or rebellion.

Considering integrity in all online representations teaches bearing accurate witness and taking responsibility for one's digital decisions and impact. Youth learn to represent truth, avoid harming others, and uphold principles even anonymously cultivating virtue that endures beyond adolescence. Wisdom also acknowledges online identities inevitably leave impressions—guiding thoughtful self-presentation avoids rash words living permanently in contextless bytes. At the same time, unrealistic social comparisons online do not undermine true worth. With compassion and consistency, diligent households impart technology's many platforms for enrichment, balanced with patience, care, and accountability wherever virtual meets reality.

Time spent immersed in digital domains undoubtedly provides value for entertainment, connection, and accessing information. However, in prioritizing endless streams of virtual engagement over enriching real-world activities, ever-present screens risk impoverishing both mind and spirit over the long term. Youth especially require varied nourishing experiences beyond what technology alone can provide for developing a virtuous, well-rounded, and content character. Though innate technology enthusiasm should not be discouraged, thoughtful families proactively foster a balanced approach integrating screen use within a life well-grounded in nature, community, and creativity. Only through cultivating diverse interests does one flourish holistically - mind, body, and social connections thriving together as an integrated whole greater than the mere sum of parts.

Uninterrupted natural contact, physical activity, and quality social interaction form crucial pillars of well-being across the human lifespan. Yet constant connectivity pulls focus inward towards individualized virtual gratification rather than the experience of life's beauty through open-hearted presence. Regular breaks from constant stimulation allow calming solitude to organize thoughts and feelings. Time invested in friendships and community fosters empathy along with confidence in navigating diverse perspectives. Creative hobbies require abstraction and problem-solving beyond what any algorithm offers. Exercise combats anxiety through endorphins while sun exposure lifts depressive symptoms. Maintaining balance honors life's richness too readily crowded out by infinite online options yet leaving one still yearning.

Families instill balance by leading by thoughtful example. Device-free family meals and vacations make present moments a priority over compulsions. Encouraging physical activities from sports to hiking nurtures wellness alongside intellectual pursuits. Exposure to art, music, and nature through hands-on creative hobbies taps hidden talents, strengthening satisfaction found within versus seeking external validation. Rather than prohibiting all virtual engagement, the structure integrates screen time within balanced schedules—making other enriching options easily accessible prevents substituting them haphazardly. Tying technology to clearly defined functions like education underscores its usefulness contributing to, not comprising, a life well lived.

Time invested face-to-face contrasts favorably with fleeting viral connections, strengthening both social skills and self-esteem derived from meaningful presence rather than superficial approvals. Building friendships requires empathy developed through reading subtleties in lived interactions unavailable online. Communities provide purpose transcending individualism by cultivating compassion through shared endeavors. Youth flourish when supported by diverse role models demonstrating virtues like diligence, integrity, and service. Drawing family closer through unplugged evenings and weekends protects against loneliness despite endless networked links. Real welfare emerges from investment in vibrant community life anchoring technology's place within it, not in isolation despite appearances of "connectedness".

Self-care encompasses diverse rejuvenating activities rediscovering life's beauty, not excessive consumption or empty pleasure-seeking. Nature walks, mindfulness meditation, journaling, and adequate rest nourish mental clarity as powerfully as nutrition sustains the body. Creative outlets aid stress management by cultivating flow states and absorbing full presence. Physical activities release feel-good endorphins balancing technology's sedentary effects, preserving health across generations to come. Achieving balance honors life's sanctity over fleeting hedonism - time invested in diversely uplifting oneself and community pays profound lifelong dividends far outweighing any momentary virtual gratification.

Rather than prohibiting interests, guidance shapes innate curiosities towards fulfillment. As interests in gaming, coding, or content creation emerge, structure explores advancing skills through moderated engagement and real-world application. Suggesting safer online communities of shared interest nurtures belonging without 24/7 dependency. Journaling progresses ideas while meditative walks incubate solutions to challenges. Developing intrinsic sources of satisfaction protects youth from relying on fickle external approval and sparks growth into independent and purposeful adults. Technology enhances well-lived lives—not defines them—when judiciously channeled towards constructive personal and social ends.

Holistic well-being emerges from diverse nourishing experiences, connections, and interests balancing screen immersion within reality - a collaborative effort of caregivers and children alike. With compassion guiding innate proclivities constructively, each generation remains empowered to reap rewards while avoiding the potential costs of extremes. Through open-hearted leadership nurturing the virtue of character, community, and purpose beyond oneself, families foster resilience for youth to thrive throughout life's unpredictable changes. Ultimately, balance considers technology enhancing lives rooted primarily in nature, creativity, and compassion - tools carefully integrated within, not substitutes for, an existence fully lived.

As we stand at the crossroads of the digital revolution and the well-being of our children, the imperative to act is clear. The challenges posed by the unchecked use of technology and social media are formidable, but with a comprehensive and proactive approach, we can transform these obstacles into opportunities for growth and empowerment.

By establishing clear boundaries, promoting responsible digital behaviors, and nurturing a balanced lifestyle, we can equip our children with the tools they need to thrive in the digital age. Through the cultivation of self-discipline, confidence, and resilience, we can empower them to navigate the complexities of the modern world with a strong sense of self, an unwavering spirit, and a deep appreciation for the richness of human connection.

As parents, educators, and caregivers, we must take a stand and become the architects of a future where our children are not merely passive consumers of technology, but rather, empowered individuals who leverage digital tools to enrich their lives, contribute to their communities, and shape a better world. It is our collective responsibility to ensure that the digital age becomes a catalyst for the holistic development of our children, fostering mental strength, self-discipline, and a profound sense of confidence and self-respect.

Together, we can cultivate a generation of mentally strong, resilient, and self-empowered individuals who will not only navigate the challenges of the present but also pave the way for a brighter, more connected future.

Disclaimer

The information provided in this book is for educational and informational purposes only. The author and publisher have made every effort to ensure that the information in this book is accurate and up-to-date at the time of publishing, but they make no representations or warranties concerning the accuracy, applicability, fitness, or completeness of the contents of this book.

The advice and strategies contained herein may not be suitable for every situation. The author and publisher disclaim any liability for any loss or damage caused by the use or misuse of the information contained in this book.

This book is not intended to replace professional advice, whether medical, legal, financial, or otherwise. If professional assistance is required, the services of a competent professional person should be sought.

The author and publisher shall not be liable for any special, incidental, consequential, or indirect damages arising directly or indirectly from the use of this book.

About the Author

Maher Asaad Baker (In Arabic: ماهر أسعد بكر), is a Syrian musician, author, journalist, VFX & graphic artist, and director. He was born in Damascus in 1977. He grew up with a dream of being one of the most well-known artists in the world, and he has been working hard to achieve it ever since.

He started his career in 1997 when he was only 20 years old. He had a passion for technology and media, and he taught himself how to develop applications and websites. He also explored various types of media-creating paths, such as music production, graphic design, video editing, animation, and filmmaking. He was not satisfied with just being a consumer of media; he wanted to be a creator of media.

Reading was another source of inspiration for him. He was always surrounded by books as a child, thanks to his father's extensive library. He read books from different genres, topics, and perspectives. He read books for knowledge, for wisdom, for entertainment, for enlightenment. Reading stimulated his imagination and curiosity. Reading also developed his writing skills.

He did not start writing professionally until later in his life, as he was busy with other projects and pursuits. But when he did start writing, he proved himself to be a talented and prolific writer. He wrote articles for various newspapers and magazines on topics such as politics, culture, society, art, technology, and more. He wrote books that were informative and insightful. He wrote books that were creative and captivating. He wrote books that were best-selling and award-winning.

He is most known for his book "How I wrote a million Wikipedia articles", where he shares his experience of being one of the most prolific contributors to the online encyclopedia. He reveals his methods, techniques, strategies, and secrets of writing high-quality articles on any subject in record time. He also discusses the benefits and challenges of being a Wikipedia editor in the age of information overload.

He is also known for his novel "Becoming the man", where he tells the story of a young man who goes through a series of transformations in his life. The novel explores themes such as identity, masculinity, self-discovery, love, loss, and redemption. The novel is based on his journey to becoming who he is today.

Copyright © 2024 Maher Asaad Baker

Cover image designed by Freepik